# Keto Bread

*The Ultimate Low-Carb Cookbook with a Mouthwatering Collection of Quick and Easy to Follow, Delicious Ketogenic Bakery Recipes to Intensify Weight Loss, Fat Burning, and Healthy Living!*

*Serena Baker*

# Table of Contents

# Introduction

Congratulations on purchasing your copy of the *"Keto Bread Cookbook"*!
I'm delighted that you have chosen to add more recipes to your Keto diet plan.

It may be surprising to an individual starting out with the Keto diet that you can still make delicious and healthy bread with just a few changes to traditional bread recipes. I am looking forward to sharing with you about the plethora of flavors and varieties of bread that can be enjoyed starting today.

While traditional breads are made with yeast and dairy products, you will find that the substitutions that are used for these keto recipes mimic the chewy and spongy that are found in original recipes. In my opinion, they taste even better and will keep you more full.

I am excited to share with you the savory and sweet varieties of keto breads to you in this cookbook. I am sure that you will prefer these breads over the recipes that you have made in the past and that you will enjoy them more as they will not kick you out of ketosis.

So let's get started on learning about and incorporating some delicious breads in your diet.

# Chapter 1: Everything You Need to Know About the Ingredients and Bread Making in the Keto Diet

## Ingredients

You will find there are several staples in the Keto diet that substitute for the old fashioned ingredients in bread-based recipes. So you have a better understanding of these new ingredients you will have in stock in your pantry, I have created a small guide to what these ingredients are and how they are helpful to your health.

### Almond flour

Almond flour is the most popular flour found in the Keto diet as an alternative to gluten-filled flours. First off, the fat content is greater than wheat flour which is a plus when following the Keto diet. As a precaution, this flour does burn much more quickly, so you need to pay close attention to your baked goods when they come close to being done. To counteract this, most recipes that include almond flour have a lower temperature setting for the stove.

Instead of buying this flour at the store, you can opt to create the same in the comfort of your own kitchen. The only ingredient is raw and unsalted almonds which are powdered over 2 to 3 minutes' time in your handy food blender. Because this flour only contains almonds, it is high in heart-healthy fats and of course, is naturally free of any gluten.

This flour is also preferred because it manages blood sugar levels beautifully and actually improves heart health. It gives you a natural boost in your energy levels which also coincides with aiding in your goal of weight loss.

If you find that you are craving your grandmother's old bread recipes, you can convert them by factoring 50% additional almond flour versus the wheat flour that was used in her recipes.

### Coconut Flour

Coconut flour has higher than normal levels of saturated fats which aid in weight loss as they improve your metabolism. This also helps to regulate your blood sugar levels in a natural way. Coconut flour is very low in sugar and carbohydrate content and very high in fiber. It even includes an enormous amount of minerals in vitamins that your body needs to keep at optimum levels.

You will find one downfall to coconut flour: it is higher in cost. However, there are smaller amounts of this flour required compared to almond flour because it has a high absorbency rating. One of the other benefits it has is that it will keep you fuller for a longer period of time and the flavor goes well with the baked Keto sweets, especially with fruits.

Because of the high fiber content which is equal to five times more than wheat flour, it aids and improves digestive health. This will also lead to weight loss, keeping you on track for your personal goals.

Just like almond flour, coconut flour gives your body the boost of energy from the high levels of medium-chain fatty acids (MCTs) that are contained within. This will certainly keep you working towards your weight loss goals.

And if that was not enough, there are antibacterial and antiviral components found in coconut flour which will keep you from getting ill and is the number one choice for the Keto lovers that have nut allergies.

## Swerve Sweetener

Swerve is one of the most popular versions of sweetener available because it balances the levels of insulin and glucose in the blood which is very beneficial for everyone, especially diabetics. The other overall benefit is that it lowers blood pressure and inflammation throughout the body. These benefits also aid the sufferers of heart diseases and weight issues.

## Erythritol Sweetener

Erythritol is also highly popular as it has many of the same benefits as Swerve sweetener. For diabetics, it enables the blood vessels to work at peak levels by leveling out the glucose in the blood stream. It has no effect on blood sugar levels or insulin production and has also found to have beneficial effects for heart patients. The common brand name of Erythritol is Stevia.

## Monks Fruit Sweetener

Monks fruit sweetener is also a popular choice which can be substituted for confectioners' sugar in any recipe. This sweetener will make your dishes sweeter versus the other choices of sweeteners. However, the people who do prefer monks fruit sweetener find that other sweeteners have a cooling effect and bad aftertaste. If you find this to be true, this will be the choice in sweeteners for you to switch to.

## Stevia Liquid Drops

This is the liquefied version of Stevia or Erythritol which packs quite a sweet taste and can be used as a confectioner sugar substitute. A little bit goes a long way as you only need 7 drops of liquid when substituting for 2 teaspoons of sweetener.

## Truvia

Truvia is the brand name for the natural sweetener of the stevia plant. Most people who are into eating healthy have heard of stevia or the common name is erythritol. This is a sugar alcohol that is found in melons and grapes and also has no calories. Many people say that there is a metallic taste to stevia, but others compare it to the same taste as traditional sugar. Again, experiment with the sweeteners to find what suits your palate.

As a note, if you have been diagnosed with autoimmune disorders or a leaky gut, it may actually have ill effects for your digestive system. If you suffer from these disorders or are allergic to corn, consult your doctor about which sweetener is best for your personal diet.

You can use granulated sweeteners in place of confectioner sweeteners. If you do substitute the granulated sweeteners, you will find that you will be able to feel the texture of the granules in your sweet treats. The confectioner sweeteners do work best in the sweet recipes, but it is up to your personal preference.

## All About Yeast

You will find that the active ingredient in any bread product is going to be the yeast. When properly activated, it will create carbon dioxide that is required for the bread to grow in size. This is due to the air pockets that are created by the carbon dioxide which are held in by the stretchy properties of the dough itself.

You cannot see it, but the carbon dioxide reproduces multiple thousands of times in each bread product. It is why the bread will grow noticeably larger in size when left to properly rise before and during baking.

Before the baking process, you will see the largest difference in the expansion of the bread. This process continues when heat is applied after the initial rising process. While the bread is baking, it permanently traps the carbon dioxide that was trapped in the dough and grows a little larger and will keep its shape after being removed from the heat.

You will find that the bread loaves will have larger air pockets in comparison to muffins. This is due to the different textures of the bread products. This is why it is harder to get bread loaves to rise versus smaller items such as biscuits and muffins.

## Dry Active Yeast

This is used in a couple of the recipes and requires the most patience. These recipes may pop out to you as they include the ingredient of honey. Before you think that I have made a mistake, honey is purposefully mixed with the yeast so that it can properly activate. The yeast requires the sugars that are present in the honey to create the needed carbon dioxide to perform the rising capabilities.

Through the baking process, this sugar is burned off, much like the process involved with cooking with alcohol. You know that the yeast is doing its job when it starts to froth in the bowl after the 7 minutes has passed for it to activate.

If you have problems with the yeast bubbling, it is due to the water not being the correct temperature. If you have the water hotter than 110° Fahrenheit, then you have actually killed the yeast preventing it from activating. If the water is cooler than 105°, then it is not hot enough to activate the yeast in the first place. Both of the results mean you need to start the process of warming the water yet again. Avoid having to repeat the steps by having a kitchen thermometer handy to ensure this finicky component will work properly. You will find that this process takes much longer than the other more common ingredient used in leavening bread.

## Baking Soda

You may remember science class where you had the replica of the volcano where you had baking soda and red food coloring inside and poured simple vinegar inside the well. Immediately the volcano erupted with all the red lava glory.

This is what is happening with your bread on a smaller and much less messy scale. As you can see from this illustration, the baking soda used in the Keto diet breads have a much quicker rising process and does not need to be monitored as in the case of the dry active yeast. This is why this is the preferred way of modern bread making.

# Chapter 2: Successful Bread Making on the Keto Diet

## Keto Bread Tips

Do not get frustrated if a dish does not turn out perfectly as you are baking with new ingredients which are usually fussy and will take some practice. However, read through these tips carefully to gain the knowledge that you will require to have your Keto breads turn out to be a success!

### *Temperature is everything*

You want to use eggs, cream cheese, sour cream, milk and any other cooled items set at room temperature. This is due to cold items not mixing particularly well into the almond and coconut flours which are used in Keto and if they are not brought down to room temperature, then your bread will not properly rise.

A trick for the eggs, in particular, is to use a bowl of warm water to immerse the eggs for the duration of 4 minutes. This will quickly bring them to room temperature which is a nice trick in case you forgot to pull them out of the fridge.

### *Make sure that you measure your ingredients properly*

This will lead to consistent results for all the Keto recipes that you find. The correct method in measuring is to spoon the ingredient into the cup rather than scooping it out of the bag directly. This will create perfect results every time as you will not over pack the ingredients using this method. You can also ensure that all the ingredients are the correct increments if you purchase a simple kitchen or baking scale.

### *Ensure the yeast is properly proofed*

Not every recipe includes dry active yeast. However, for the ones that do, there is a specific process to follow as outlined in those particular recipes. It includes combining the yeast with honey for the yeast to feed upon. Do not worry about the sugar content as the honey is for the yeast to feed upon, creating the carbon dioxide required for the bread to rise. The sugar will be cooked off during the process and will not be present in the final result.

Once combined, you will blend water which is the specific temperature of 105° - 110° which can be checked with a kitchen thermometer or it will be slightly warm to the touch. You will know that this process was successful by the mixture becoming bubbly after waiting for a period of 7 minutes.

If there are no bubbles, simply repeat the process with the correct temperature water. You will not waste a whole dish because this occurs at the beginning of the recipe.

### Again, temperature is important during the rising process

You want to keep your rising bread in an environment where the temperature is not going to vary much and will be undisturbed during the rising time. You want to have the area to be slightly warm and humid, but not hot as this will stop the rising process. It is suggested to keep the covered tray on top of the stove which is preheating.

### Keep away from xylitol

When using any yeast in your recipes, you want to make sure that xylitol is not an additive in your ingredients as it rapidly decreases the rising of the dough and will cause them to become flat. You will find that Monk Fruit and Erythritol do not contain xylitol and may be used as a substitute for sweeteners that have this additive included.

### Loaf pan size is important

There are a wide variety of baking pans out there. I have made it easy by including the particular pan that is required for each recipe. However, if you do not have that specific size, always opt to go with a pan that is the next size up rather than downsizing. This will ensure that the dough will not rise too far causing the bread to burst over the pan.

The measurements for pans are calculated from the top of the pan and does not include the pan itself. The following is an easy guide for the standard size of loaf pans:

- 2 cups of bread (mini loaf pan) - 5 3/4" x 3 1/4" x 2"
- 3 cups of bread - 7 3/8" x 3 5/8" x 2"
- 4 cups of bread - 8" x 4" x 2 1/2"
- 6 cups of bread - 8 1/2" x 4 1/2" x 2 1/2"
- 8 cups of bread - 9 1/4" x 5 1/4" x 2 1/2"

### Pure ingredients are everything

Especially when dealing with the different varieties of cheese, you want to make sure there are no preservatives or additives. Also, opt for the skim or whole milk types as these will have less water to weep during the baking process.

When baking powder is being used, it is a priority to ensure that it is as fresh as possible. Since there is no gluten present, it needs to be of the best quality to make the rising process work properly.

Not sure if your baking powder is still active? Do a small test by combining with boiling water. If bubbles occur immediately, then your baking powder will make your bread properly rise.

### A perfect way to grease any pan

If you want to make sure that you do not run into the problem of your Keto breads sticking to the pan, this fail-proof trick will take the headache out of baking. Dissolve 2 teaspoons of coconut oil in a saucepan and then apply to your pan with a pastry brush. Set in the freezer for a minimum of 20 minutes as the oil hardens. Pull out of the freezer before filling with your dough.

### Separating the eggs is a necessary step

It may seem like a pain at the time, but there is a reason that you will find the eggs are separated. This simple measure also helps the Keto breads to rise. When incorporating the whipped eggs into the batter, do not over mix. This is due to you counteracting the airiness that has been created by whipping the eggs and your breads will not rise properly.

### For the bread loaves

If you find that your bread is crumbling when you are slicing, ensure the loaf is completely cooled. This will help the bread to set and firm up more when given the time to come to room temperature.

### For the muffins

If you are having trouble with your muffins rising properly, add a combination of baking soda and vinegar which causes the carbon dioxide reaction required for proper rising. You will also find that many of the recipes already incorporate this trick.

### Tips for the cookies

Different people enjoy cookies hard or soft. Luckily there is a trick in Keto baking which lets you have a choice. The biggest trick is to have the treats completely cool so that the cookie will not crumble.

If you like to have softer cookies, leave them on the countertop in a lidded container or cookie jar. They will keep fresh for up to 5 days. Refrigerate the cookies after they are completely cooled in a covered tub and they will become harder. They will keep for up to 7 days this way.

If your cookies are not rising the way you prefer, simply combine a half teaspoon of apple cider vinegar while blending the batter. You will find some of the recipes already utilize this trick.

### For the Bagels:

Coconut creates bagels that are denser. On the other hand, almond flour creates a light bagel. You can substitute whichever flour for the result that you prefer.

# Nutritional Information Note for this cookbook

Nutritional information for the recipes provided is an approximate only. And substitutions that you use will alter the nutritional values and need to be personally researched to stay on track with the Keto diet. As such, I cannot guarantee the complete accuracy of the nutritional information given for any recipe in this cookbook. Erythritol carbs are not included in the net carb counts as it has been shown not to impact blood sugar.

# Chapter 3: Bread Loaf Recipes

## Cauliflower Bread Loaf

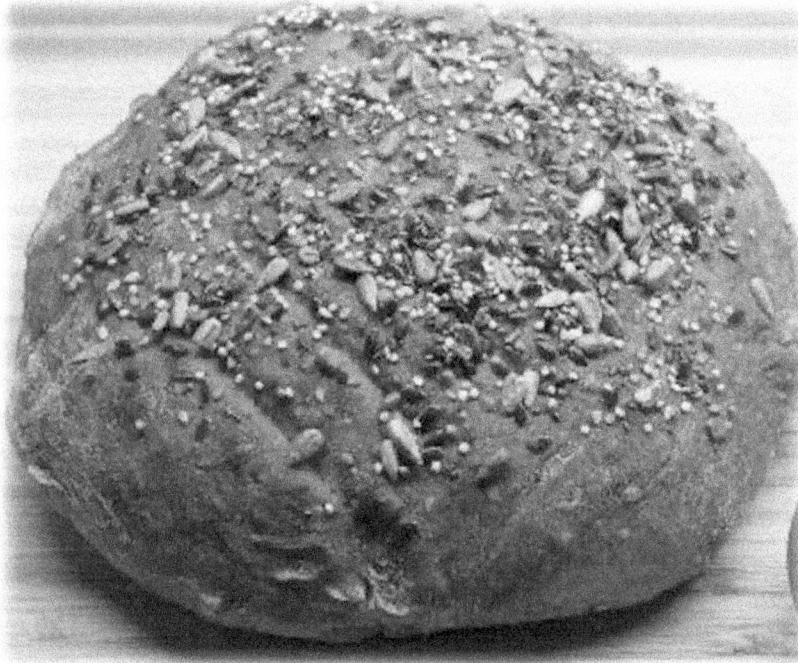

Total Prep & Cooking Time: 30 minutes
Level: Intermediate
Makes: 12 Slices
Nutritional information per slice:
Protein: 4 grams
Net Carbs: 3 grams
Fat: 4 grams
Sugar: 0 grams
Calories: 90

### What you need:

- 0.5 tsp. salt
- 2 cups almond flour
- 1.5 tsp. sesame seeds
- 0.25 cup psyllium husk
- 2 cups cauliflower florets

- 1.5 tsp. pumpkin seeds
- 5 large eggs, beaten
- 0.5 tsp. baking soda
- coconut oil cooking spray
- 1.5 tsp. sunflower seeds
- 3 tsp. coconut oil
- Medium skillet
- 8 x 4-inch bread loaf pan

**Steps:**

1. Divide the cauliflower into pieces and transfer to a food blender. Pulse for about 1 minute until the consistency is crumbly.
2. Warm the cauliflower in a frypan with the coconut oil for approximately 5 minutes as it becomes soft. Remove from the burner.
3. Distribute the cauliflower into a kitchen towel and wring to eliminate the extra moisture. Repeat this step as many times as necessary to ensure the liquid has been eliminated. Put to the side.
4. Set your stove to the temperature of 350° Fahrenheit.
5. Cover the pan completely with baking lining and coat with the coconut oil on the base and sides. Set to the side.
6. Whip the eggs in a glass dish and blend the baking soda, psyllium husk, and almond flour until integrated.
7. Gently toss the riced cauliflower into the batter until it is a smooth consistency.
8. Distribute into the prepped pan and use a scraper to ensure it is even throughout.
9. Evenly dust the sunflower, sesame, and pumpkin seeds on the dough.
10. Warm for approximately 55 minutes and transfer to the countertop.
11. Transfer to a wire rack by pulling on the baking lining.
12. Wait about 15 minutes before slicing. Enjoy!

Expert Tips:
- If you are crunched for time, you can use prepackaged riced cauliflower and use 1 cup in this recipe. This will eliminate steps 1 through 3.
- Riced cauliflower is a brilliant substitute for any recipe that calls for rice.

# Cream Cheese Bread Loaf

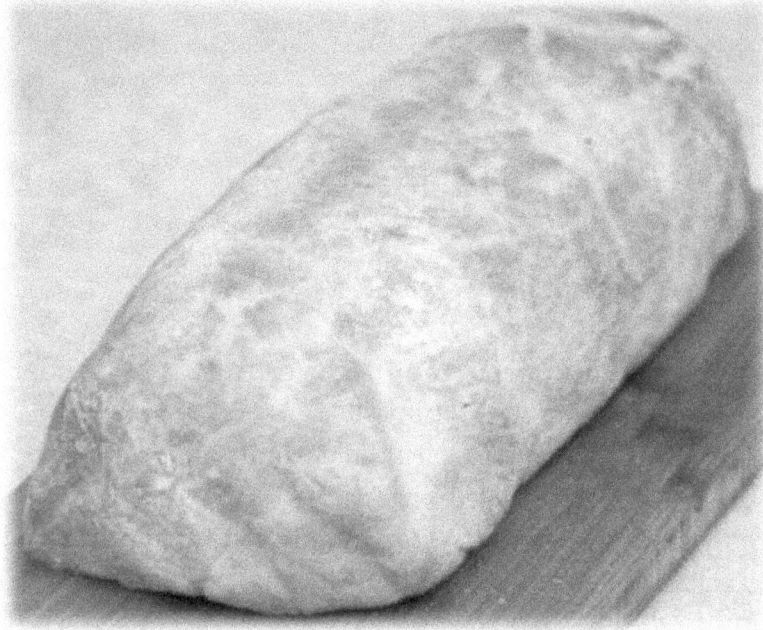

Total Prep & Cooking Time: 40 minutes / 100 minutes (See Expert Tip Below)
Level: Beginner
Makes: 12 Slices
Nutritional information per slice:
Protein: 6 grams
Net Carbs: 1.6 grams
Fat: 19 grams
Sugar: 0 grams
Calories: 204

## What you need:

- 8 large eggs
- 8 oz. cream cheese, full-fat and softened
- 0.5 cup butter, unsalted and softened
- 1.5 cups coconut flour
- 0.5 cup sour cream, full-fat
- 4 tsp. baking powder, gluten-free
- 1 tsp. salt
- 3 tsp. butter, unsalted and separated
- 1 tbsp. Swerve sweetener, granulated

- food blender
- 12 cavity muffin tin or 9 x 5 inch bread loaf pan (See Expert Tips below)

**Steps:**

1. Ensure your butter, cream cheese, and eggs are not cold. Do not skip this step.
2. Set the stove to heat at the temperature of 350° Fahrenheit.
3. Smear one tbsp. of butter on the baking pan and set to the side.
4. Completely blend the Swerve, salt, baking powder, and coconut flour in a glass dish with a whisk to dispel any lumpiness.
5. Use a food blender to pulse the room temperature cream cheese and leftover butter until light for approximately 60 seconds, removing the excess from the sides of the bowl during the process.
6. Blend one egg in the food blender until integrated while continuing to ensure the ingredients are scraped from the edges. Repeat for the leftover eggs until complete.
7. Gently distribute the flour dish to the blender while pulsing on the lowest setting until incorporated fully.
8. Finally, stop pulsing the dough and toss the sour cream in the dish without over mixing.
9. Distribute the batter to the prepped pan and press with a scraper to ensure it is even throughout.
10. Heat for a total of 1 hour and check on the loaf. If not complete, continue to heat at 10-minute intervals until a utensil comes out without residue. It should take no more than 90 minutes in total.

Expert Tips:
- Alternatively, this recipe can be made into 12 muffins. Be sure to use butter liberally on the tin. The cooking time is diminished to half an hour.
- If you prefer to enjoy your bread without a touch of sweetness, the Swerve can be eliminated from the recipe.

# Garlic Cheese Bread Loaf

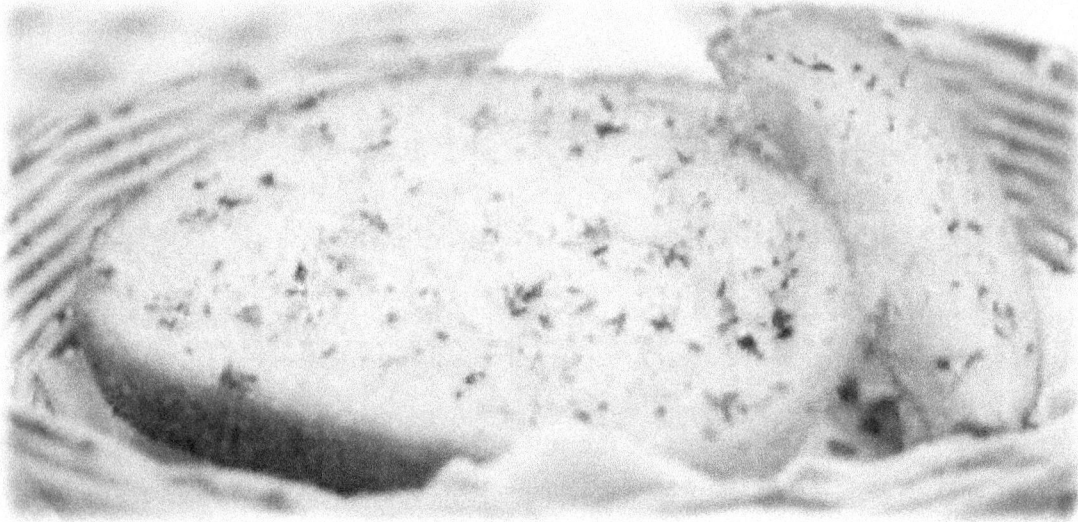

Total Prep & Cooking Time: 30 minutes
Level: Beginner
Makes: 10 Slices
Nutritional information per slice:
Protein: 11 grams
Net Carbs: 4 grams
Fat: 27 grams
Sugar: 0 grams
Calories: 299

## What you need:

- 1 tbsp. parsley seasoning
- 0.5 cup butter, unsalted and softened
- 2 tbsp. garlic powder
- 6 large eggs
- 0.5 tbsp. oregano seasoning
- 1 tsp. baking powder, gluten-free
- 2 cup almond flour
- 0.5 tsp. xanthan gum
- 1 cup cheddar cheese, shredded
- 0.5 tsp. salt
- food blender

- 9 x 5 inch bread loaf pan

**Steps:**

1. Set your stove to heat at the temperature of 355° Fahrenheit.
2. Utilize baking lining to cover the pan and set to the side.
3. Use a food blender to pulse the eggs until smooth. Combine the butter and pulse for an additional 60 seconds until integrated.
4. Blend the almond flour and baking powder for approximately 90 more seconds until the batter thickens.
5. Finally combine the oregano, garlic, parsley, and cheese until integrated.
6. Distribute into the prepped pan and smooth evenly with a scraper.
7. For approximately 45 minutes, heat the bread and check with a utensil to ensure it has baked properly when it comes out without residue.
8. Transfer to the countertop and wait about 15 minutes before slicing and serving.

# Herbed Bread Loaf

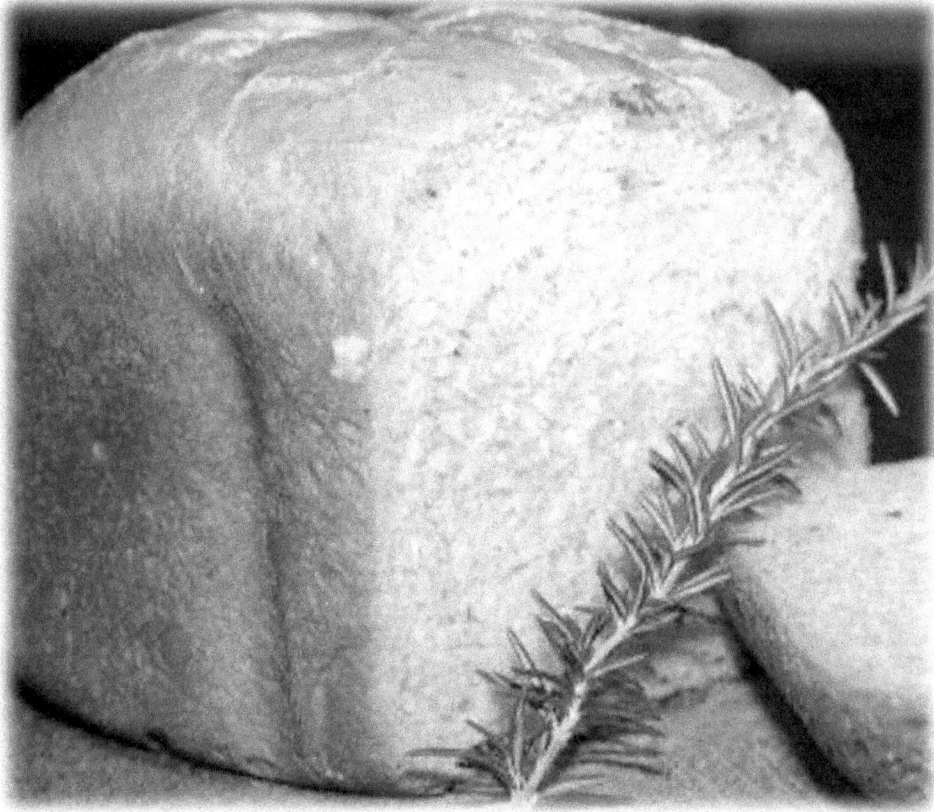

Total Prep & Cooking Time: 45 minutes / 60 minutes
Level: Beginner
Makes: 12 Slices
Nutritional information per slice:
Protein: 6 grams
Net Carbs: 0.5 grams
Fat: 10 grams
Sugar: 1 gram
Calories: 127

## What you need:

- 2.5 cups almond flour
- 8 oz. cream cheese, full-fat
- 1.5 tsp. baking powder, gluten-free
- 0.25 cup coconut flour

- 0.5 cup butter, unsalted
- 1 tsp. rosemary seasoning
- 8 whole eggs
- 1 tsp. sage seasoning
- 2 tbsp. parsley seasoning
- 3 tsp. butter, unsalted and separate
- food blender
- 3 mini loaf pans or an 8 x 4 inch bread loaf pan

## Steps:

1. Heat the stove at a temperature of 350° Fahrenheit.
2. Prepare your choice of pan(s) thoroughly with one tbsp. of butter and set to the side.
3. Blend the cream cheese and the leftover 1/2 cup of butter in a food blender for approximately 45 seconds until the consistency is smooth.
4. Combine the parsley, sage, and rosemary into the blender and pulse for another half minute until integrated.
5. Whip one egg in the blender until combined. Repeat for the other 7 eggs until complete.
6. Finally, blend the coconut flour, baking powder, and almond flour for an additional 90 seconds until the batter is a thick consistency.
7. Distribute to the prepped pan(s) evenly while smoothing with a scraper.
8. If using the mini pans, heat for 35 minutes. Increase the timing to 50 minutes if using the large pan.
9. Utilize a utensil to see if any residue remains after poking into the center.
10. Transfer to the countertop and wait approximately 15 minutes before dividing and serving.

# Lemon Bread Loaf

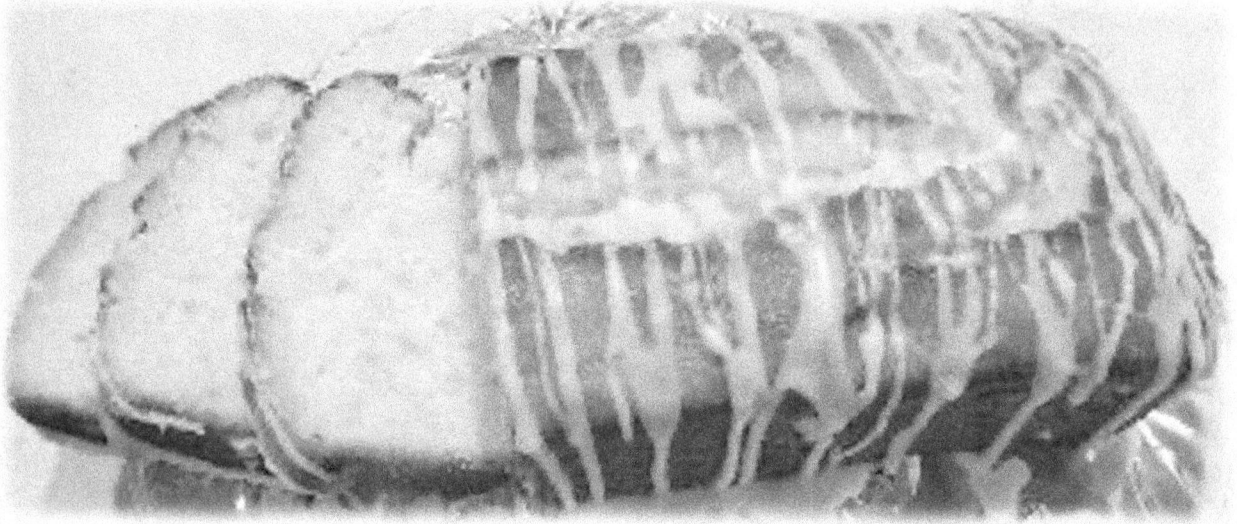

Total Prep & Cooking Time: 70 minutes
Level: Beginner
Makes: 15 Slices
Nutritional information per slice:
Protein: 3 grams
Net Carbs: 2 grams
Fat: 10 grams
Sugar: 0 grams
Calories: 121

## What you need:

*For the bread:*

- 6 large eggs
- 10 tbsp. coconut flour
- 9 tbsp. butter, melted and cooled
- 2 tbsp. cream cheese, full-fat and softened
- 1.5 tsp. baking powder, gluten-free
- 1 tsp. vanilla extract, sugar-free
- 2 tbsp. heavy whipping cream
- 0.67 cup Swerve sweetener, granulated
- 0.5 tsp. salt
- 2 tbsp. lemon zest

- 4 tsp. lemon juice
- saucepan
- food blender or electric blender
- 8 x 4 inch bread loaf pan

*For the topping:*

- 1 tsp. lemon zest
- 2 tbsp. Swerve sweetener, confectioner
- 3 tsp. heavy whipping cream
- 2 tsp. lemon juice

## Steps:

1. Dissolve the butter in a saucepan and remove from the burner. Set to the side.
2. Adjust the stove to the temperature of 325° Fahrenheit.
3. Use an electric blender or food blender to pulse the baking powder, salt, heavy whipping cream, Swerve, salt, and cream cheese for approximately 2 minutes until fully integrated.
4. Empty the butter, lemon juice, coconut flour, and lemon zest to the mixture and blend until incorporated.
5. Distribute the batter to the prepped pan. Press the top with a scraper to ensure it is the same thickness throughout.
6. Heat for a total of 55 minutes in the stove.
7. In the meantime, blend the lemon juice, heavy whipping cream, Swerve, and lemon zest for approximately 60 seconds until the consistency is smooth.
8. Check the loaf with a utensil to make sure no residue is present once pulled out of the center.
9. Move to the countertop and flip on a cake platter to separate the bread from the pan and wait about 10 minutes.
10. Spread the glaze completely over the bread. It will drip down to the plate.
11. Slice and serve at your desired temperature. Enjoy!

# Pumpkin Bread Loaf

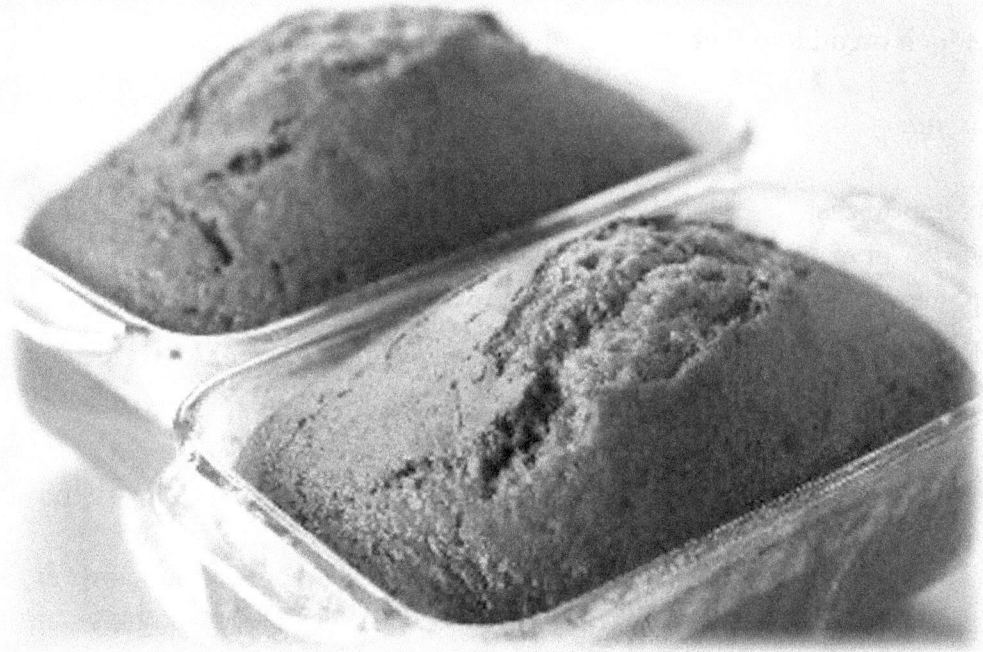

Total Prep & Cooking Time: 40 minutes / 65 minutes
Level: Beginner
Makes: 12 Slices
Nutritional information per slice:
Protein: 4 grams
Net Carbs: 0.8 grams
Fat: 9 grams
Sugar: 0 grams
Calories: 172

## What you need:

- 0.5 cup almond flour, blanched
- 2 tbsp. coconut flour
- 0.25 cup Truvia
- 0.5 tbsp. baking powder, gluten-free
- 3 large eggs, beaten
- 0.5 tsp. pumpkin spice seasoning
- 0.125 tsp. salt
- 0.5 tbsp. coconut oil
- 3 tbsp. butter, unsalted

- 0.125 cup pumpkin puree
- 0.5 tsp. vanilla extract, sugar-free
- 4 mini loaf pans or a 9 x 5 inch bread loaf pan

## Steps:

1. Heat your stove at the temperature of 350° Fahrenheit.
2. Use baking lining to layer over your choice of pan(s) and set to the side.
3. Use a glass dish to blend the almond flour, Truvia, baking powder, and coconut flour, whisking to remove any lumpiness.
4. In an additional dish, integrate the coconut oil and butter. Nuke for about half a minute in the microwave.
5. Blend the eggs, vanilla extract and pumpkin puree to the butter until combined well.
6. Incorporate the flour into the mixture until the consistency is smooth.
7. Evenly distribute into your preferred baking pan.
8. Heat in the stove for a total of 30 minutes for the mini pans and 55 minutes for the large pan.
9. Distribute to the countertop and wait approximately 15 minutes before sectioning into individual slices and serving.

# White Bread Loaf

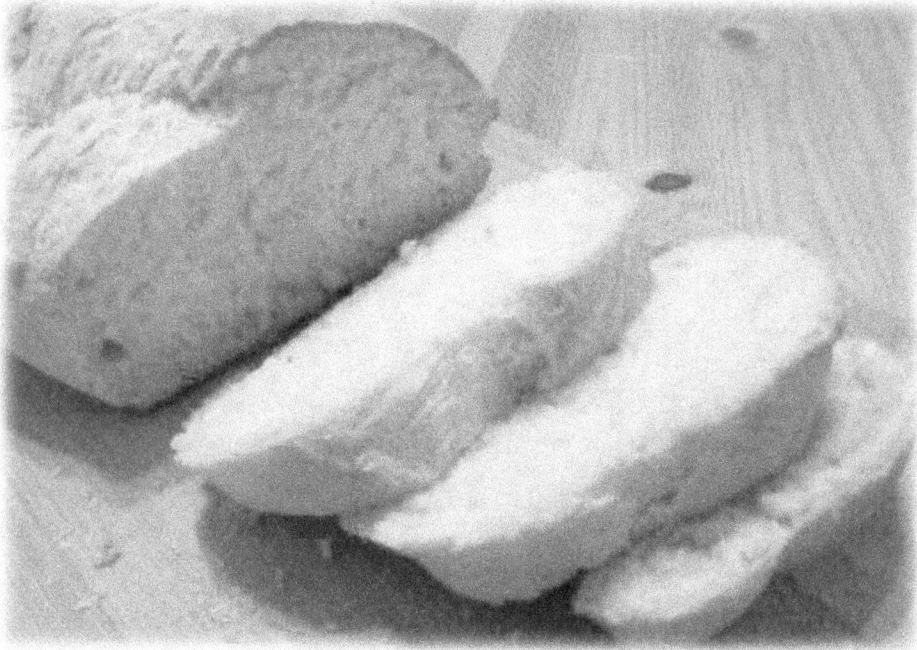

Total Prep & Cooking Time: 70 minutes
Level: Beginner
Makes: 15 Slices
Nutritional information per slice:
Protein: 6 gm
Net Carbs: 3 gm
Fat: 14 gm
Sugar: 0 gm
Calories: 167

## What you need:

- 1.5 tsp. baking powder, gluten-free
- 5 large eggs, whites and yolks separated
- 2.5 cups almond flour, blanched and sifted
- 0.33 cup coconut flour, sifted
- 0.25 cup butter, melted and cooled
- 0.5 tsp xanthan gum
- 0.25 tsp. salt
- 0.67 cup almond milk
- 0.25 tsp. cream of tartar

- saucepan
- electric blender
- 9×5 inch loaf pan

## Steps:

1. Ensure the eggs and butter are at room temperature before starting. Do not skip this step.
2. Liquefy the butter using a saucepan and remove from the burner. Set aside.
3. Adjust the temperature of the stove to heat at 350° Fahrenheit.
4. Cover the pan with a layer of baking lining and set to the side.
5. Use an electric blender to pulse the egg yolks for approximately 3 minutes and then blend the butter until incorporated.
6. Blend the almond flour, xanthan gum, baking powder, salt, milk, and coconut flour for about 2 minutes until integrated fully.
7. In a separate dish, use an electric blender to blend the cream of tartar and egg whites for approximately 4 minutes until stiffened.
8. Use a rubber scraper to combine the egg whites into the batter making sure not to over mix.
9. Distribute into the prepped pan and use a rubber scraper to smooth and press the batter evenly.
10. Warm for approximately 55 minutes or until a utensil is poked into the center and removed without residue.
11. Distribute to the countertop and wait for about 10 minutes.
12. Flip the bread onto a platter and wait another 5 minutes before slicing. Enjoy!

Expert Tips:
- This bread loaf keeps fresh for 7 days if stored in a lidded container in the refrigerator.
- Feel free to substitute coconut oil in place of the butter.
- If you would like to have a mounded bread loaf, opt for the 8 x 4-inch pan.
- You can top with any seasoning you would like before baking if you want to get creative with the flavors.

# Chapter 4: Bun and Roll Recipes

## Bacon & Cheese Rolls

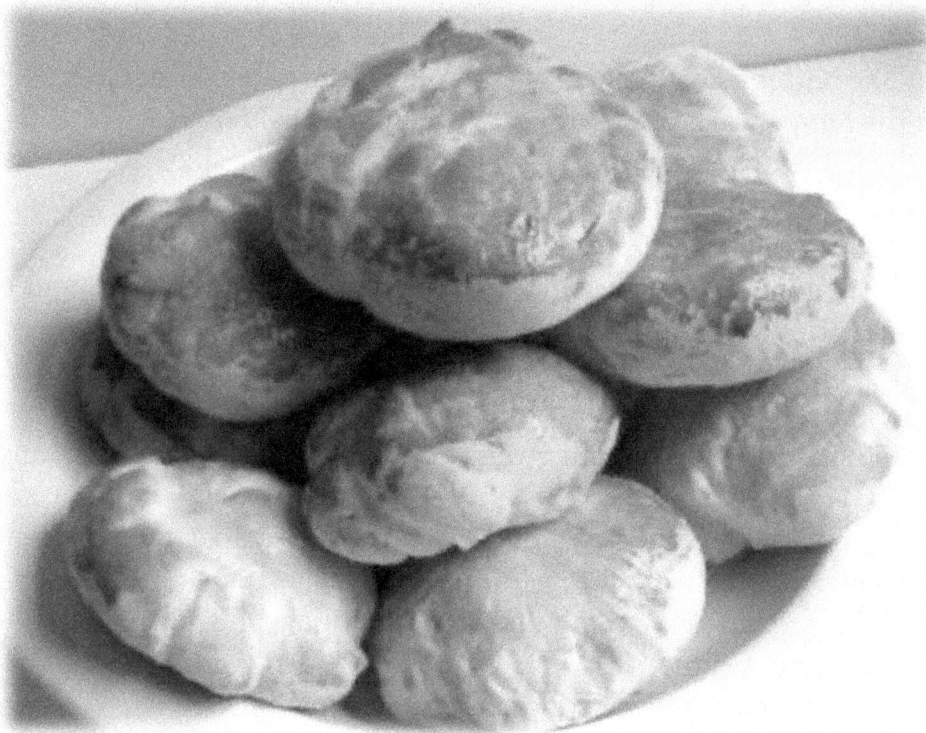

Total Prep & Cooking Time: 40 minutes
Level: Beginner
Makes: 12 Rolls
Nutritional information per roll:
Protein: 9 grams
Net Carbs: 0 grams
Fat: 12 grams
Sugar: 0 grams
Calories: 149

### What you need:

- 0.5 cup mozzarella cheese, grated
- 5 oz. bacon, uncooked and diced
- 2 tbsp. cream cheese, full-fat

- 0.5 tsp. black pepper
- 2 tbsp. sesame seeds
- 1 tbsp. psyllium husk
- 1 cup cheddar cheese, grated
- 3 large eggs
- 1.5 tsp. baking powder, gluten-free
- 0.25 tsp. salt
- medium skillet
- food blender
- standard sized flat sheet

**Steps:**

1. Set your stove to heat at the temperature of 355° Fahrenheit.
2. Layer baking lining on the flat sheet and set aside.
3. Brown the bacon in a frypan for approximately 5 minutes and take away from the burner.
4. Blend the cream cheese to the pan and set to the side for another 5 minutes.
5. Combine the mozzarella cheese, black pepper, sesame seeds, psyllium husk, cheddar cheese, eggs, baking powder, and salt into a food blender.
6. Empty the bacon mixture into the food blender and pulse for approximately 4 minutes until integrated fully.
7. Distribute the batter into 12 mounds on the prepped flat sheet and heat for about 15 minutes.
8. Serve hot and enjoy!

Expert Tips:
- These rolls can be stored in a plastic bag in the fridge for 5 days.
- You can also use this recipe to make 24 mini muffins if you prefer. Follow the same instructions.

# Butter Croissants

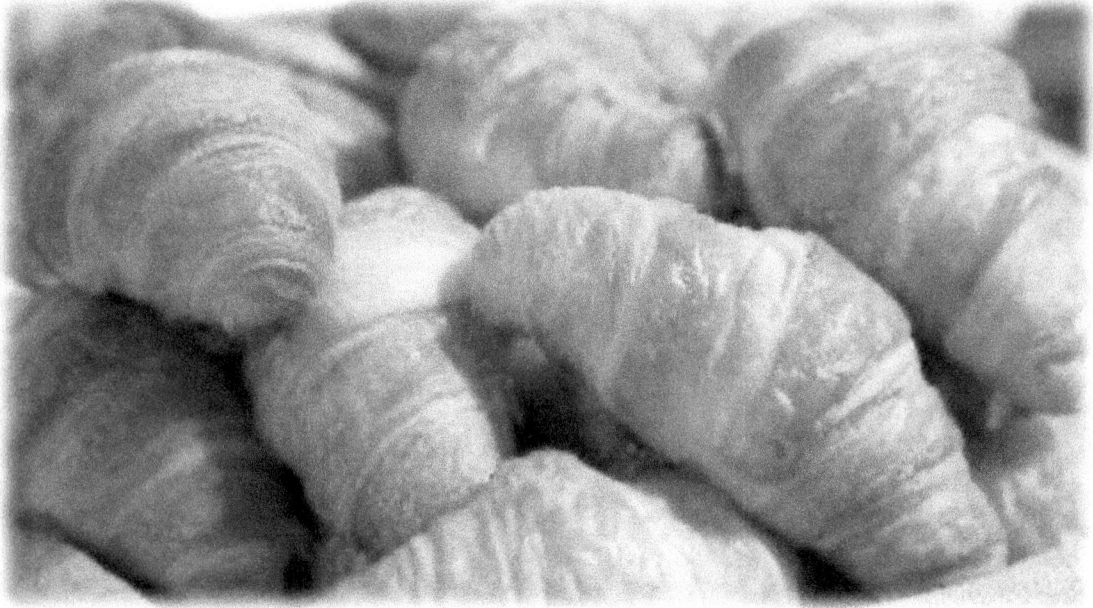

Total Prep & Cooking Time: 60 minutes
Level: Beginner
Makes: 6 Croissants
Nutritional information per croissant:
Protein: 9 grams
Net Carbs: 1.4 grams
Fat: 9 grams
Sugar: 1 grams
Calories: 124

## What you need:

- 4 egg whites
- 0.25 tsp. cream of tartar
- 1 tsp. Mrs. Dash, original
- 3 tsp. mayonnaise, sugar-free
- 1 cup cheddar cheese, shredded
- 3 egg yolks
- food blender
- standard sized flat sheet

**Steps:**

1. Heat your stove to the temperature of 300° Fahrenheit.
2. Prepare the flat sheet by covering with baking lining. Set to the side.
3. Use a food blender or electric blender to combine the cream of tartar and egg whites for approximately 4 minutes until stiffened.
4. In an additional dish, blend the cheddar cheese, Mrs. Dash, mayonnaise and egg yolks until well-integrated.
5. Fully incorporate the mixtures together and make sure not to overmix.
6. Form long mounds by dropping with a large spoon onto the prepped flat sheet.
7. Heat for 35 minutes in the stove and turn the stove off.
8. Keep the croissants in the oven for about 5 more minutes and then transfer to a wire rack.
9. Wait about 10 minutes before serving and enjoy!

# Cloud Bread

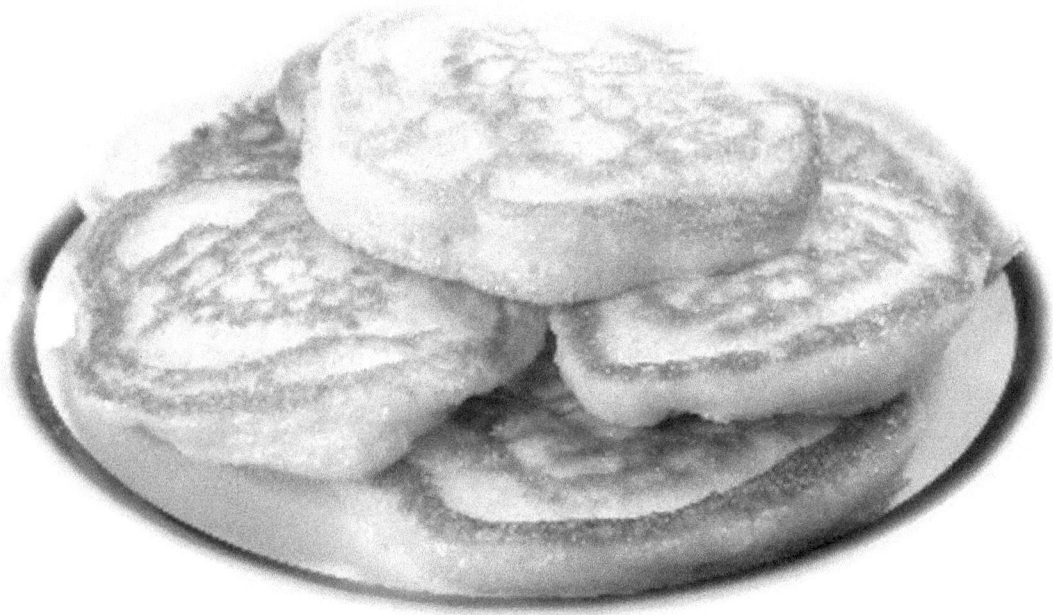

Total Prep & Cooking Time: 40 minutes
Level: Beginner
Makes: 6 Helpings
Nutritional information per piece:
Protein: 4 grams
Net Carbs: 0.6 grams
Fat: 7 grams
Sugar: 0 grams
Calories: 85

## What you need:

- 3 oz. cream cheese, full-fat and softened
- 0.125 tsp. salt
- 3 large eggs
- 0.25 tsp. cream of tartar
- electric blender
- standard sized flat sheet

## Steps:

1. Adjust the temperature of the stove to heat at 300° Fahrenheit.
2. Layer a flat sheet with baking lining and set to the side.

3. Divide the whites and yolks of the eggs into two different dishes.
4. Blend the salt and cream cheese with the yolks with an electric blender.
5. Combine the cream of tartar with the whites of the eggs and pulse with the electric blender for approximately 4 minutes until firm.
6. Blend the two dishes together and be sure not to over mix.
7. Evenly distribute the batter into 6 sections on the prepped flat sheet.

8. Slightly press each mound to flatten to your desired thickness.
9. Heat for approximately half an hour and distribute to a wire rack.
10. Enjoy immediately with a half tbsp. of butter.

# Dinner Rolls

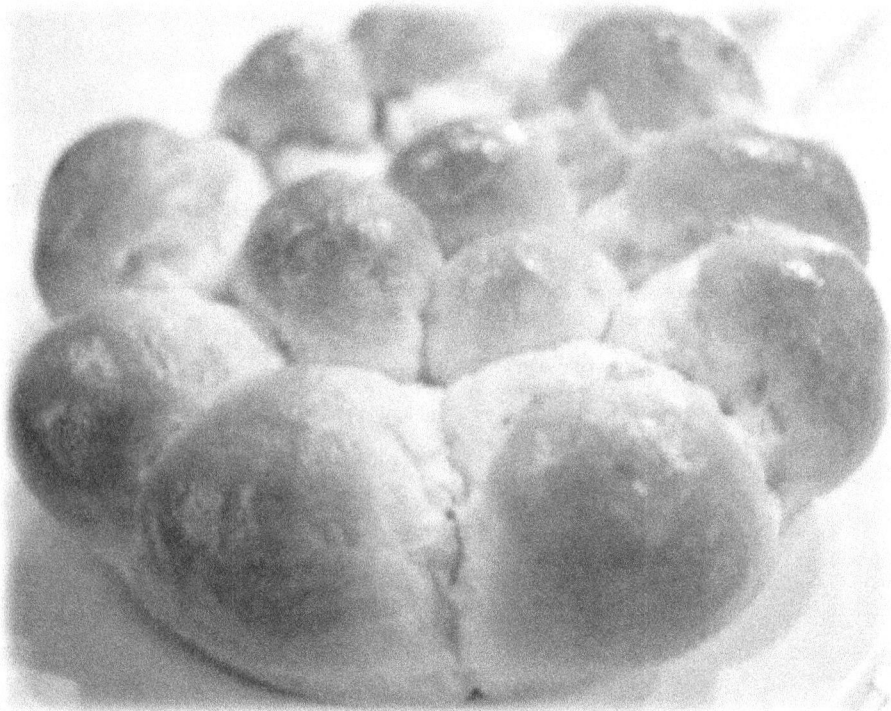

Total Prep & Cooking Time: 45 minutes
Level: Beginner
Makes: 12 Rolls, 2 rolls per helping
Nutritional information per helping:
Protein: 13 grams
Net Carbs: 1.1 grams
Fat: 19 grams
Sugar: 1 grams
Calories: 234


## What you need:

- 8 oz. cream cheese block, full-fat
- 1 tbsp. butter, unsalted
- 3 cups mozzarella cheese, shredded and whole-milk
- 4 large eggs
- 1.33 cups almond flour
- 4 tbsp. baking powder, gluten-free
- medium saucepan
- large cast iron skillet

**Steps:**

- Set your stove to heat at the temperature of 400° Fahrenheit.
- Use a saucepan to warm the mozzarella and cream cheese together over the lowest setting for approximately 2 minutes while constantly tossing.
- Transfer the cheese to a glass dish and combine with the eggs, almond flour, and baking powder for about 90 seconds until the consistency is smooth.
- Wait about 15 minutes before dividing into 12 sections.
- Create mounds from each section and distribute to a plate.
- Refrigerate for about 10 minutes.
- Dissolve the butter in a cast iron skillet over the lowest heat setting.
- Arrange the mounds so that they are touching in the skillet and heat for approximately 20 minutes until they puff up and turn golden.
- Serve immediately and enjoy!

Expert Tips:

- If you find the dough is too sticky to form into mounds, place the dough in the fridge for 10 minutes prior to creating the balls as well as after.
- To help your rolls to properly rise, make sure you are using fresh baking powder and ingredients without preservatives or additives.

# Garlic Rolls

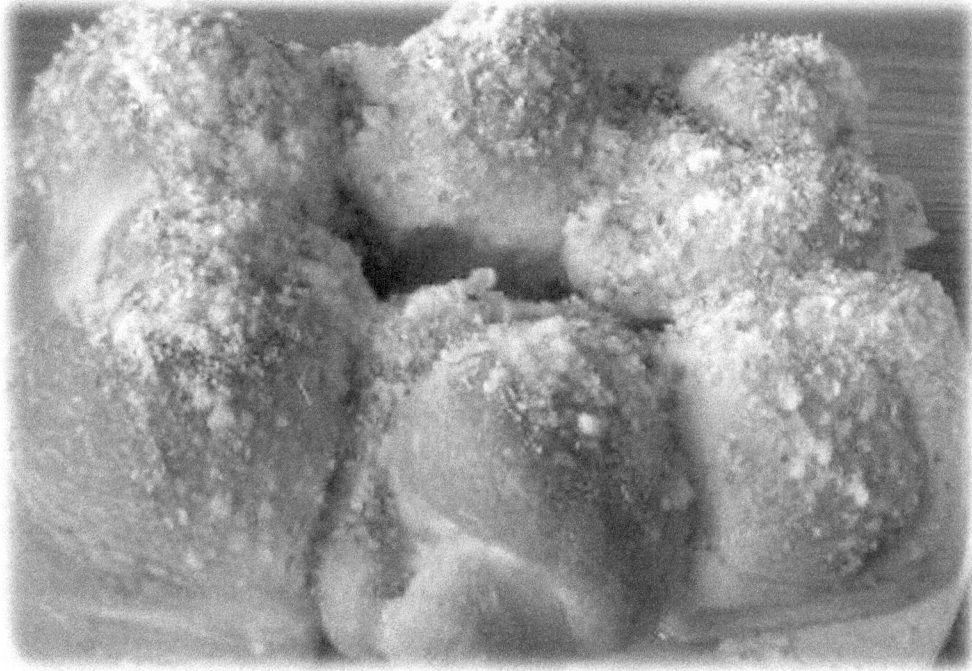

Total Prep & Cooking Time: 35 minutes
Level: Beginner/Intermediate
Makes: 6 Rolls
Nutritional information per roll:
Protein: 17 grams
Net Carbs: 3 grams
Fat: 26 grams
Sugar: 1 gram
Calories: 310

## What you need:

- 0.5 cup parsley, chopped
- 2.5 cups mozzarella cheese, shredded
- 1.5 cups almond flour, blanched
- 2 oz. cream cheese, full-fat
- 0.67 cup parmesan cheese, grated and separated
- 3 large eggs
- 1 tsp. baking powder, gluten-free
- 0.33 cup bacon, uncooked
- 4 garlic cloves, minced finely

- 1 tsp. Italian seasoning
- 0.25 cup butter, unsalted and melted
- coconut oil cooking spray
- large cast iron skillet
- medium saucepan
- additional large skillet

## Steps:

1. Coat a frypan with the cooking spray and brown the bacon until your desired crispiness. Set on a kitchen paper covered plate and set to the side.
2. Coat the skillet with the cooking spray and set aside.
3. In a microwave-safe dish, nuke the cream and mozzarella cheese for 60 seconds.
4. Combine the melted cheese, eggs, baking powder, and almond flour and crush the cooked bacon into small sections. Incorporate well.
5. Blend the Italian seasoning and 1/2 cup of the parmesan cheese in a separate glass dish.
6. Spoon the mixture and form into 6 individual mounds.
7. Rotate the balls in the Italian seasoning and transfer to the prepped skillet.
8. Dust with the leftover 1/8 cup of parmesan cheese and refrigerate for 10 minutes.
9. Adjust your stove to heat at the temperature of 400° Fahrenheit.
10. Place the skillet into the stove and heat for approximately 22 minutes.
11. In the meantime, dissolve the butter and garlic in a frypan.
12. When the rolls have puffed up and turned golden, transfer to the countertop.
13. Brush the garlic butter over the top and serve immediately.

# Ham & Cheese Rolls

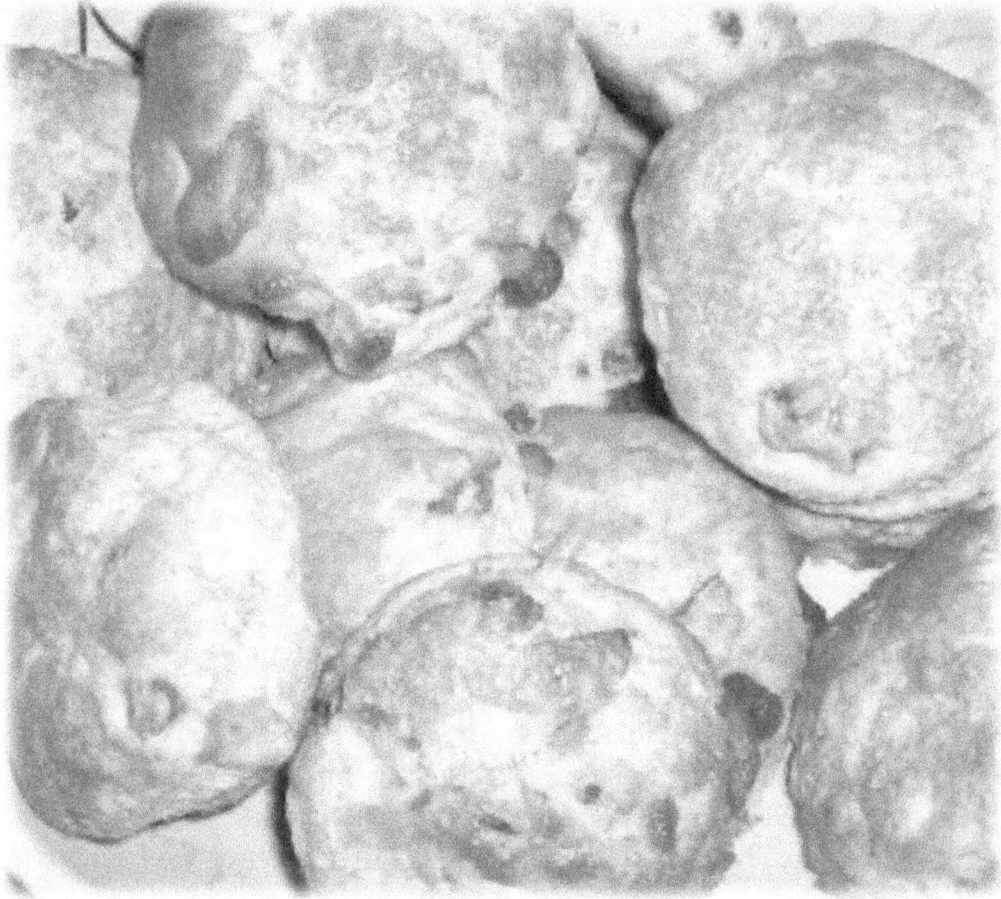

Total Prep & Cooking Time: 20 minutes
Level: Beginner
Makes: 6 Rolls
Nutritional information per roll:
Protein: 17 grams
Net Carbs: 3 grams
Fat: 13 grams
Sugar: 1 gram
Calories: 198

## What you need:

- 0.5 cup cheddar cheese, shredded
- 1 cup deli ham, diced
- 0.75 cup mozzarella cheese, shredded
- 2 large eggs

- 0.5 cup parmesan cheese, grated
- standard sized flat sheet

**Steps:**

1. Heat the stove to the temperature of 375° Fahrenheit. Prepare a flat sheet with a layer of baking lining.

2. Blend the diced ham, eggs, mozzarella, and cheddar cheese in a glass dish until integrated well.
3. Divide the batter into 6 equal sections and create mounds. Transfer to the prepped flat sheet.
4. Heat for approximately 18 minutes in the stove until they turn slightly golden.
5. Enjoy immediately.

Expert Tips:
- You can also use this recipe to create muffins or a variation of cloud bread.
- Get creative with the cheese and substitute any dry and hard variety.

# Hamburger Buns

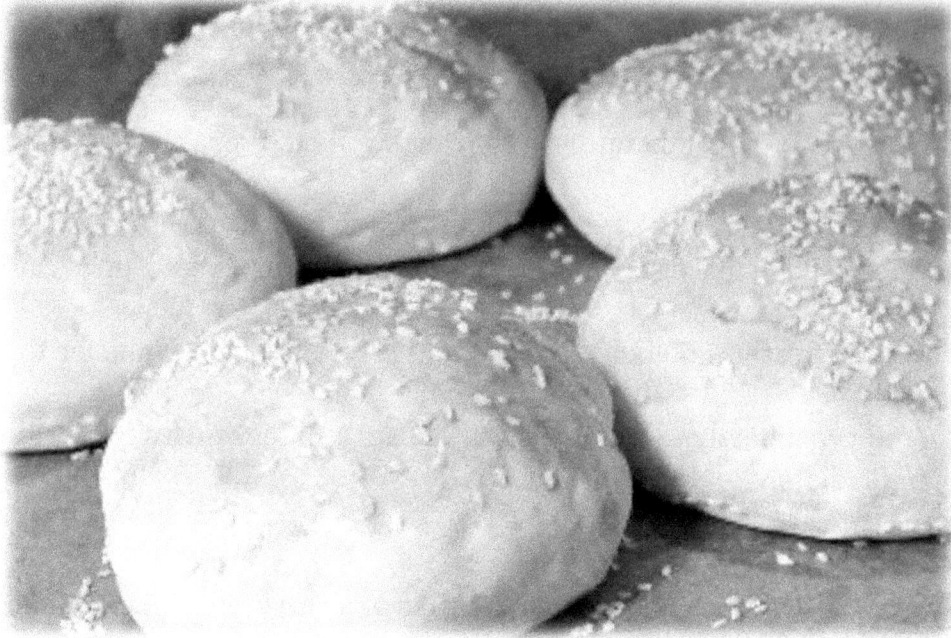

Total Prep & Cooking Time: 120 minutes
Level: Intermediate/Expert
Makes: 6 Buns
Nutritional information per bun:
Protein: 8 grams
Net Carbs: 3 grams
Fat: 22 grams
Sugar: 1 gram
Calories: 262

## What you need:

- 1 tbsp. apple cider vinegar
- 2 tsp. active dry yeast
- 0.25 tsp. cream of tartar
- 2 tsp. honey (See Expert Tips below)
- 0.5 cup lukewarm water
- 0.25 cup butter, unsalted, melted and cooled
- 2 tsp. xanthan gum
- 1.33 cup almond flour
- 0.67 cup golden flaxseed meal, ground finely
- 0.125 cup whey protein isolate

- 2 tsp. baking powder, gluten-free
- 0.125 cup psyllium husk, ground finely
- 1 tsp. salt
- 3 egg whites, room temperature
- 0.25 tsp. ground ginger
- 1 large egg, room temperature
- 0.25 cup sour cream, room temperature
- coconut oil cooking spray
- medium saucepan
- standard sized flat sheet

**Steps:**

1. Pulse the flaxseed meal and psyllium husk in a food blender for approximately 2 minutes as they become a fine powder. Set aside.
2. Use a saucepan to warm the water to approximately 105° Fahrenheit.
3. In the meantime, prepare a flat sheet by covering with a layer of baking lining. Set to the side on top of the stove.
4. Blend the honey and yeast in a glass dish. Empty the lukewarm water into the yeast and use a kitchen towel to lay over the bowl.
5. Dissolve the butter in the same saucepan and turn the burner off when complete. Set to the side.
6. Let the dish rest for 7 minutes as it becomes bubbly.
7. Meanwhile, combine the ginger, cream of tartar, salt, baking powder, xanthan gum, psyllium husk, whey protein powder, flaxseed meal, and almond flour whisking to remove all lumpiness present. Set aside.
8. Once the yeast has bubbled up, blend the egg, vinegar, melted butter, and egg whites with an electric blender for approximately 2 minutes.
9. Empty half of the flour mixture into the dish and pulse for about 60 seconds.
10. Then combine 1/8 cup of the sour cream into the mixture and beat for about half a minute.
11. Blend the leftover flour mixture over about 60 seconds time and finally pulse the leftover 1/8 cup of sour cream into the batter until it thickens.
12. Slightly wet your hands and section the dough into 6 portions. Create mounds out of each section and transfer to the prepped flat sheet on the stove.
13. Apply a small amount of coconut oil spray on each and layer with a section of plastic wrap.
14. Place a kitchen towel over the buns and leave for approximately 45 minutes as they rise.
15. Check to see if the bread has properly risen. If not, leave for an additional 15 minutes until they have increased substantially.

16. Approximately 20 minutes before the time is up for the bread to rise, set your stove to heat at the temperature of 350° Fahrenheit.
17. Once the rolls have risen, discard the plastic wrap and warm in the stove for about 10 minutes.
18. Section a large piece of tin foil to place over the buns. Be sure it is not directly resting on the buns.
19. Heat for approximately 15 minutes longer and transfer to the countertop.
20. Wait about 15 minutes if you want hot buns or half an hour for room temperature buns.

Expert Tips:
- During step 5, it is imperative that the yeast becomes bubbly. This shows that the yeast has been properly activated. If not, start over again and be sure the temperature of the water is between 105° and 110° Fahrenheit. Otherwise, the yeast will not properly activate.
- Do not worry about the maple syrup not being part of the Keto diet. It is simply to activate the yeast and all the sugar will be burned off during the cooking process.
- During step 12, the buns are rising on top of the stove so that they are slightly warm during the process which helps them to rise.
- These buns will keep fresh up to 5 days when kept on the counter in a lidded tub or individually wrapped in plastic wrap.
- If you do not have xanthan gum, you can substitute 4 additional tsp. of ground flaxseed meal.
- Alternatively, you can substitute 2 tsp. of apple cider vinegar and coconut cream in place of the sour cream.

# Seeded Buns

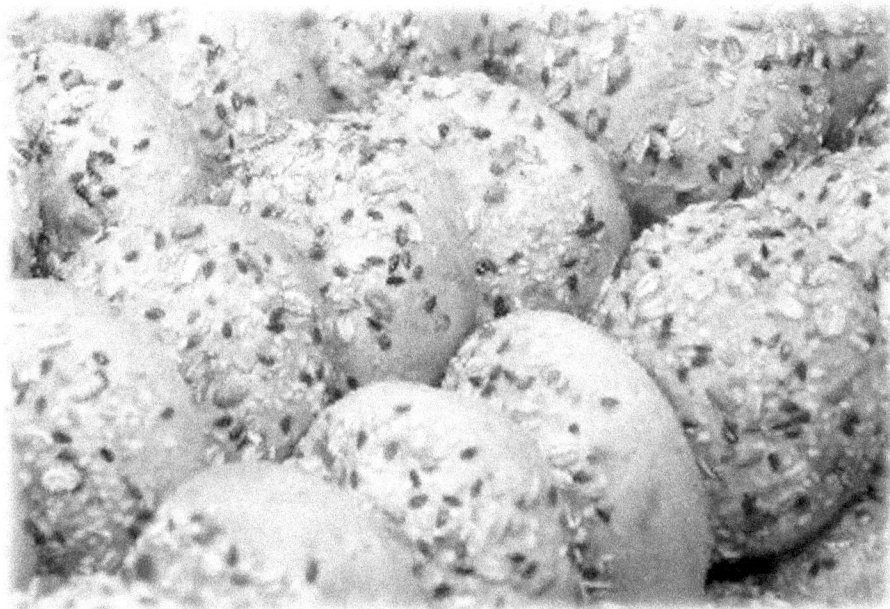

Total Prep & Cooking Time: 75 minutes
Level: Beginner
Makes: 6 Buns
Nutritional information per bun:
Protein: 3 gm
Net Carbs: 3 gm
Fat: 3 gm
Sugar: 0 gm
Calories: 73

## What you need:

- 1 cup almond flour
- 2 tsp. baking powder
- 3 egg whites
- 1.25 cup hot water
- 2 tbsp. sesame seeds or seeds of your choice
- 5 tbsp. psyllium husk powder
- 1 tsp. salt
- 2 tsp. apple cider vinegar
- medium saucepan
- standard sized flat sheet

**Steps:**

1. Warm the water in a saucepan until it starts to bubble. Transfer to a glass dish.
2. In the meantime, prepare a flat sheet with a layer of baking lining and set to the side.
3. Blend the water with the almond flour, baking powder, psyllium husk, salt, and apple cider vinegar until it becomes a thick consistency.
4. Section into 6 equal portions and form mounds.
5. Apply pressure to flatten the mounds to approximately 1 inch thick.
6. Arrange on the prepped flat sheet and glaze with the melted butter.
7. Dust with the sesame seeds and heat for approximately 35 minutes.
8. Serve immediately and enjoy!

Expert Tip:

- Get creative with the herbs and seeds that you add to this recipe. The possibilities are endless.
- Do not be alarmed if the buns turn out tinted slightly purple. This is due to the psyllium husk powder, but the bread still tastes amazing. If this puts you off, you can substitute xanthan gum in its place.

# Slider Buns

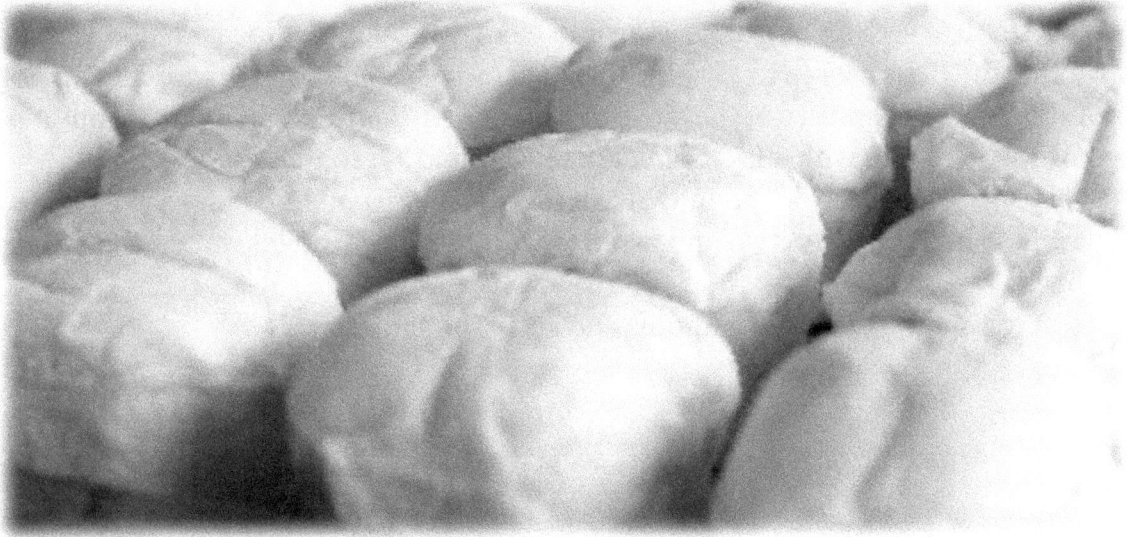

Total Prep & Cooking Time: 50 minutes
Level: Beginner
Makes: 8 buns
Nutritional information per bun:
Protein: 7 grams
Net Carbs: 2.3 grams
Fat: 13 grams
Sugar: 0 grams
Calories: 160

## What you need:

- 0.75 cup mozzarella cheese, shredded and whole milk
- 1 large egg, beaten
- 0.33 cup almond flour
- 2 oz. cream cheese, full-fat
- 0.25 tsp garlic powder
- 2 tsp baking powder, gluten-free
- 0.5 cup cheddar cheese, shredded
- standard sized flat sheet

## Steps:

1. In a microwave-safe dish, nuke the mozzarella and cream cheese for approximately 60 seconds until liquefied.

2. In the meantime, whip the eggs in another glass bowl until smooth.
3. Combine the cheese mixture, eggs, cheddar cheese, garlic powder, and baking powder and knead until the consistency becomes thick.
4. Transfer to a section of plastic wrap and empty the almond flour on top.
5. Rotate the plastic wrap to form a large ball and place in the fridge for half an hour.
6. Adjust the temperature of the stove to heat at 425° Fahrenheit about 15 minutes later.
7. Cover a flat sheet with a layer of baking lining and set to the side.
8. Once set, section the dough into quarters and create a mound from each.
9. Divide the mound into two and arrange with the sliced side down on the prepped flat sheet.
10. Heat for approximately 11 minutes and serve immediately.

# Southern Style Biscuits

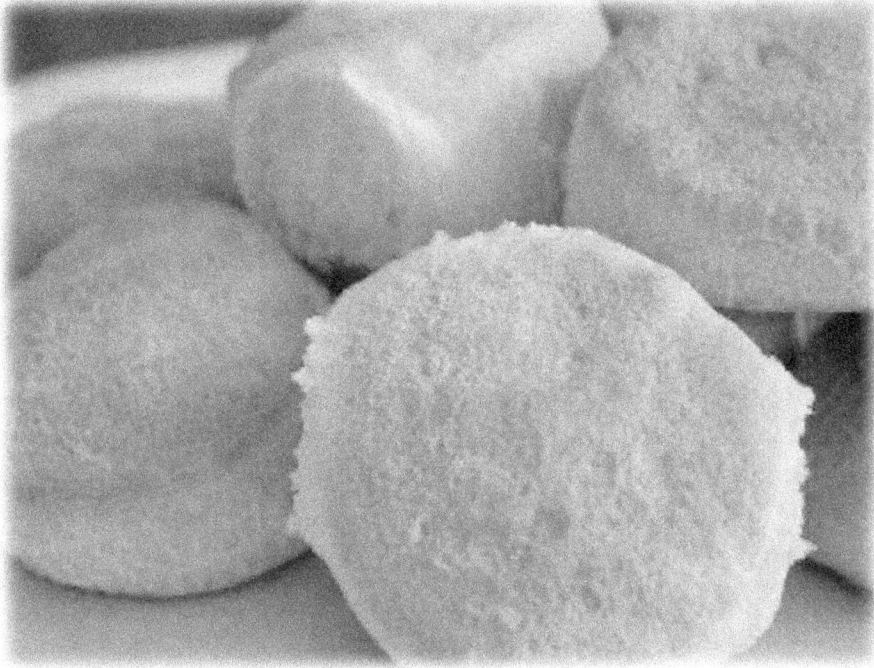

Total Prep & Cooking Time: 25 minutes
Level: Beginner
Makes: 6 Biscuits
Nutritional information per biscuit:
Protein: 16 grams
Net Carbs: 2 grams
Fat: 27 grams
Sugar: 1 gram
Calories: 330

## What you need:

- 0.75 cup almond flour, sifted
- 0.25 cup coconut flour, sifted
- 2 oz. almond milk
- 1 tsp. baking powder, gluten-free
- 3 tbsp. butter, separated
- 0.25 tsp. salt
- 5 large egg whites
- food blender or electric blender
- medium saucepan

- standard sized flat sheet

## Steps:

1. Set the temperature of the stove to heat at 400° Fahrenheit.
2. Layer baking lining on a flat sheet and set to the side.
3. Blend the almond flour, 2 tbsp. of the butter, salt, almond milk, baking powder, and coconut flour until integrated.
4. Use a food blender or electric blender to pulse the eggs for approximately 3 minutes until the stiffen.
5. Carefully blend the eggs with the batter and do not over mix.
6. Set the batter to the side for about 5 minutes as it thickens.
7. In the meantime, liquefy the leftover tbsp. of butter in a saucepan.
8. Allow dough to sit for five minutes as the coconut flour will absorb liquid.
9. Spoon the batter onto the prepped flat sheet leaving about an inch between.
10. Apply the melted butter to the top and heat in the stove for 10 minutes.
11. Enjoy while hot!

Expert Tips:
- After step 6, you want the dough to be thick and not watery. If you find that it is too watery, blend 1 tbsp. of coconut flour and wait 3 minutes. Repeat as needed for the correct consistency.
- Be sure to use non-packaged egg whites for this recipe as they will be airier.
- Ghee can be replaced for the butter. You can substitute any milk except for coconut milk as well.

# Spicy Cheddar Biscuits

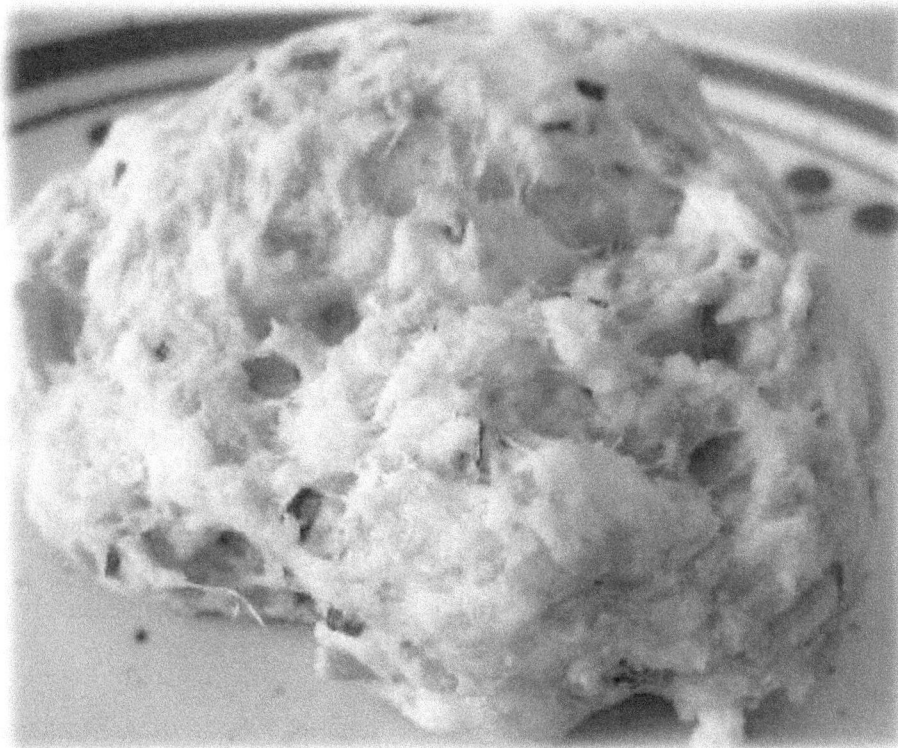

Total Prep & Cooking Time: 30 minutes
Level: Beginner
Makes: 8 Biscuits
Nutritional information per biscuit:
Protein: 9 grams
Net Carbs: 3.3 grams
Fat: 26 grams
Sugar: 0 grams
Calories: 280

## What you need:

- 2 tsp. baking powder, gluten-free
- 0.25 tsp. salt
- 2 cup almond flour
- 1 large egg
- 4 tbsp. butter, unsalted and cubed
- 0.67 cup cheddar cheese, shredded
- 3 tsp. parsley seasoning

- 0.33 cup jalapeno, diced
- 0.125 tsp. black pepper
- 0.125 cup heavy cream
- standard sized flat sheet

## Steps:

1. Heat your stove to the temperature of 350° Fahrenheit. Prepare the flat sheet with a layer of baking lining. Set to the side.
2. Blend the pepper, baking powder, cubed butter, almond flour, and salt in a glass dish with a whisk to remove all lumpiness.
3. Combine the egg and heavy cream into the mixture until incorporated.
4. Divide the jalapeno in half and discard the seeds. Chop into small chunks.
5. Transfer to the mix along with the parsley and cheddar cheese and toss until integrated.
6. Divide the batter into 6 equal portions and form mounds from each. Arrange on the prepped sheet with about 2 inches in between.
7. For approximately 18 minutes, heat in the stove and enjoy immediately.

Expert Tips:
- Get creative with the combinations in these biscuits. Other ingredients that would go well are bacon and cheese, blueberries or feta cheese and spinach.
- You can easily leave the jalapeno pepper out of this recipe if you do not prefer spicy food.

# Chapter 5: Muffin Recipes

## Banana Bread Muffins

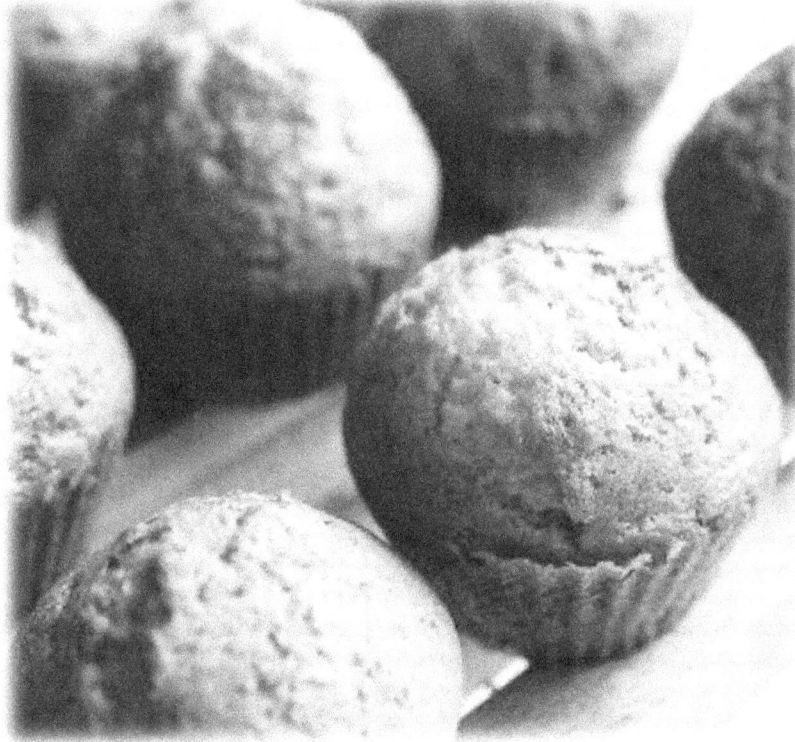

Total Prep & Cooking Time: 60 minutes
Level: Beginner
Makes: 6 Muffins
Nutritional information per muffin:
Protein: 7 gram
Net Carbs: 4 grams
Fat: 14 grams
Sugar: 1 gram
Calories: 184

### What you need:

- 0.125 cup Erythritol sweetener, confectioner
- 0.75 cup almond flour
- 1.25 tbsp. ground flax

- 3 tbsp. butter, unsalted and melted
- 0.125 cup sour cream, full-fat
- 1.25 tsp. baking powder, gluten-free
- 4 oz. walnuts, raw and chopped
- 0.33 tsp. ground cinnamon
- 2 tsp. butter, unsalted, cubed and separate
- 1.5 tsp. banana extract, sugar-free
- 2 tsp. almond flour, separate
- 0.125 cup almond milk, unsweetened
- 1 tsp. vanilla extract, sugar-free
- 2 tsp. Erythritol sweetener, confectioner and separate
- 1 large egg
- medium saucepan
- food processor
- 6 cavity cupcake tin

## Steps:

1. Dissolve the 3 tsp. of butter completely in a saucepan and set to the side.
2. Adjust the temperature of the stove to heat at 350° Fahrenheit.
3. Line a small cupcake tin with 6 papers or silicone cups. Set aside.
4. Use a food blender to pulse the 2 tsp. of almond flour, 2 tsp. of butter and walnuts until a crumbly consistency. Set to the side.
5. Blend the 1/3 cup of Erythritol, cinnamon, baking powder and 3/4 cup of almond flour until incorporated fully.
6. Combine the eggs, sour cream, banana extract, almond milk, melted butter, and vanilla extract into the mixture until integrated.
7. Evenly distribute to the prepped cupcake tin and dust with the crumble from the food processor. Apply slight pressure to adhere to the batter.
8. Evenly spread the 2 tsp. of Erythritol over the muffins.
9. Heat for a total of 20 minutes and take out of the stove to the countertop.
10. Wait about half an hour before serving. Enjoy!

Expert Tip:
- If you do not have ground flax on hand, you can take this out of the recipe.

# Cinnamon Muffins

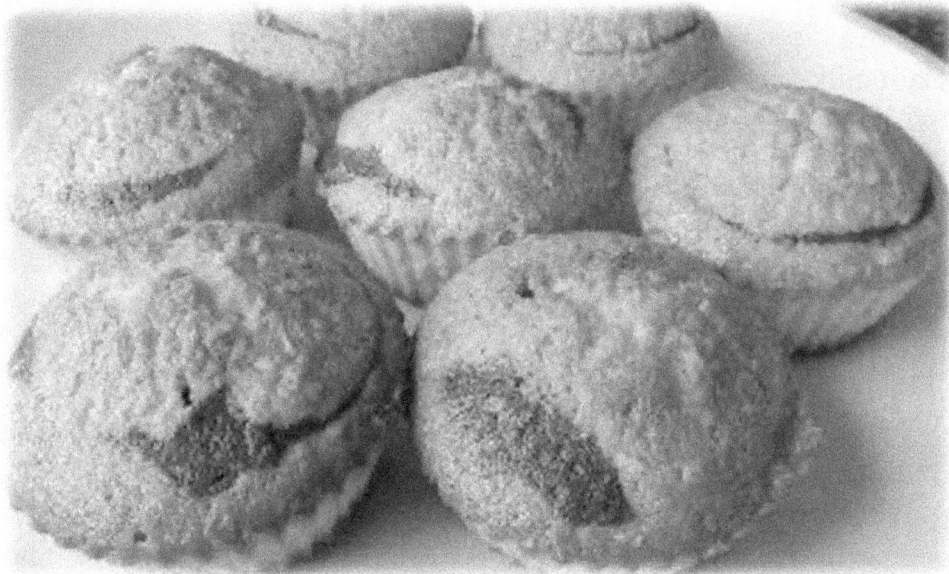

Total Prep & Cooking Time: 25 minutes / 55 minutes
Level: Beginner
Makes: 12 Muffins
Nutritional information per muffin:
Protein: 5 grams
Net Carbs: 1.8 grams
Fat: 9 grams
Sugar: 1 gram
Calories: 89

## What you need:

*For the muffin:*

- 0.33 cup almond flour
- 0.5 tsp. baking powder, gluten-free
- 0.33 cup almond butter
- 0.5 tbsp. ground cinnamon
- 5 oz. pumpkin puree
- 0.33 cup coconut oil
- 12 cavity muffin tin or 24 cavity mini muffin tin

*For the optional topping:*

- 0.125 cup coconut butter
- 0.5 tbsp. Swerve sweetener, granulated
- 0.125 cup milk
- 1.25 tsp. lemon juice

## Steps:

1. Set your stove to heat at the temperature of 350° Fahrenheit.
2. Use silicone or baking cups to line your preferred cupcake tin. Set to the side.
3. Combine the almond flour, baking powder, and cinnamon with a whisk in a glass dish. Remove any lumpiness present.
4. Blend the almond butter, pumpkin puree, and coconut oil into the mix until incorporated.
5. Evenly divide the batter between the cavities in the prepped cupcake tin.
6. Heat for approximately 13 minutes and transfer to a wire rack after waiting 5 minutes.
7. If you are applying the topping, blend the lemon juice, milk, Swerve, and coconut butter until smooth.
8. Evenly empty the topping once the muffins have completely cooled.

Expert Tips:
- If there are any leftovers, they will keep fresh for 2 days if stored in a lidded tub on the counter.
- If you need them to keep longer, wrap each in saran wrap and use a freezer-safe plastic bag to keep frozen for up to 2 weeks.
- You can substitute any seed or nut butter you wish in this recipe.
- If you do not have pumpkin puree on hand, you can easily substitute the same amount of overripe banana or unsweetened applesauce.

# Chocolate Muffins

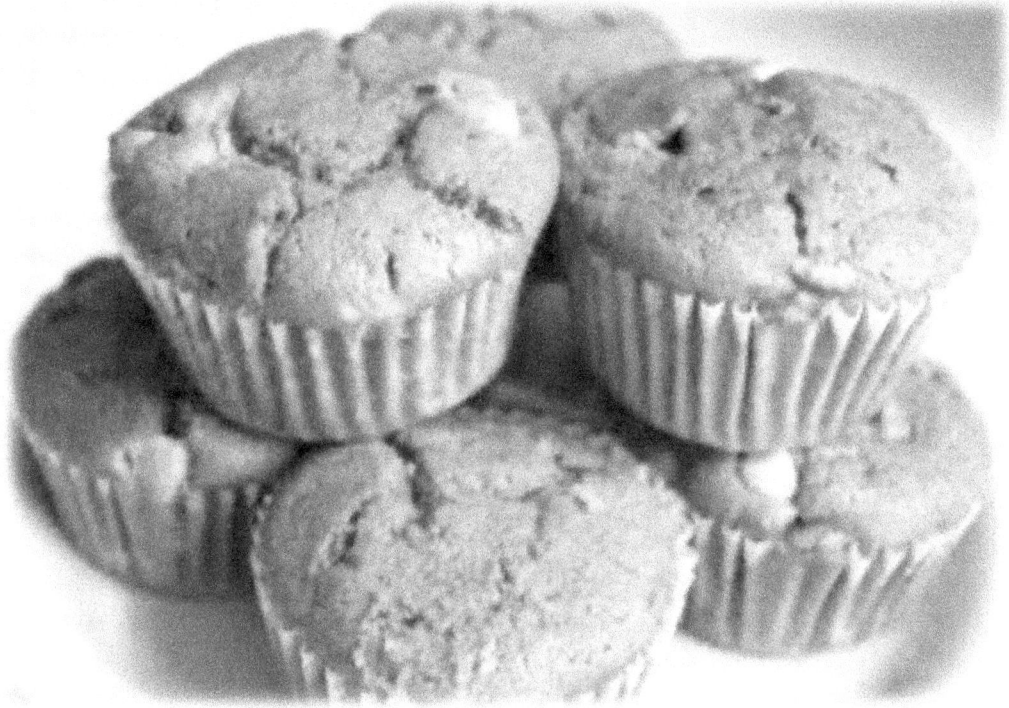

Total Prep & Cooking Time: 45 minutes
Level: Beginner
Makes: 12 Muffins
Nutritional information per muffin:
Protein: 7 grams
Net Carbs: 3.5 grams
Fat: 16 grams
Sugar: 1 gram
Calories: 189

## What you need:

- 0.5 tsp. salt
- 2 cups almond flour, blanched
- 0.5 cup cocoa powder, unsweetened
- 0.75 cup Pyure Stevia blend, granulated
- 1 tsp. baking powder, gluten-free
- 4 large eggs
- 0.25 cup coconut oil, melted
- 2 oz. almond milk, unsweetened

- 1 tsp. vanilla extract, sugar-free
- 1.75 oz. dark chocolate, Stevia sweetened and chopped
- medium saucepan
- 12 cavity muffin tin

## Steps:

1. Set the temperature of the stove to heat at 350° Fahrenheit. Cover the cavities of the cupcake tin with baking liner or silicone. Set to the side.
2. Liquefy the coconut oil for approximately 3 minutes in a saucepan.
3. Chop the chocolate roughly into small chunks and set aside.
4. Blend the salt, baking powder, almond flour, Pyure Stevia blend, and cocoa powder until fully incorporated.
5. Combine the melted coconut oil, vanilla extract, almond milk, and eggs into the mix and toss until integrated.
6. Finally, incorporate the chopped chocolate into the mix.
7. Evenly divide the batter to the prepped cupcake tin.
8. For the duration of approximately 26 minutes, heat the muffins and then transfer to the countertop.
9. Wait about 10 minutes before serving and enjoy!

# Coffee Cake Muffins

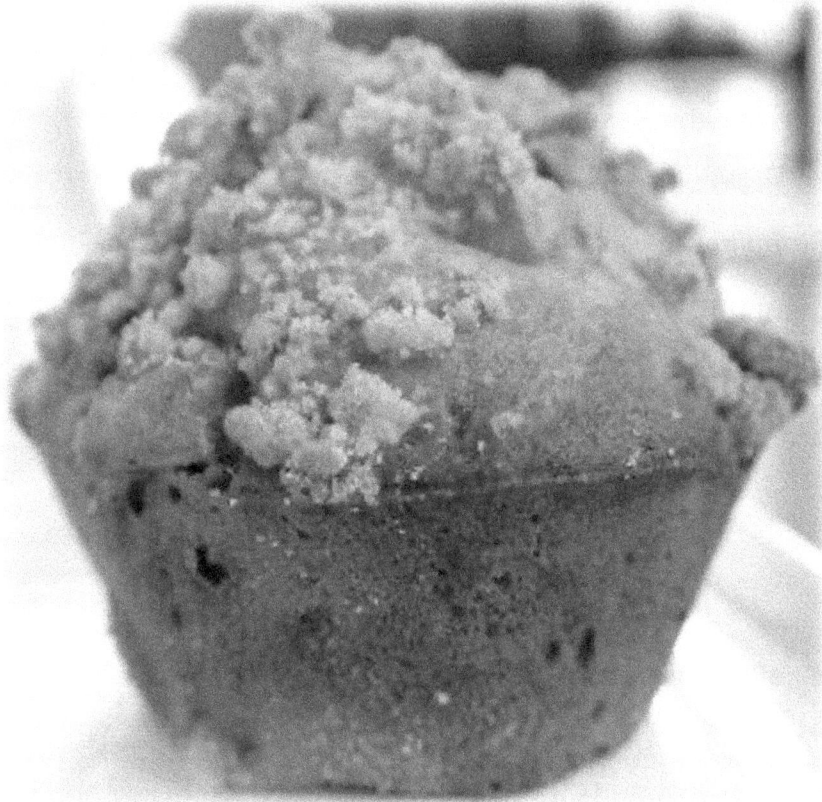

Total Prep & Cooking Time: 35 minutes /45 minutes
Level: Beginner
Makes: 12 Muffins
Nutritional information per muffin:
Protein: 9 grams
Net Carbs: 3.9 grams
Fat: 24 grams
Sugar: 1 gram
Calories: 284

## What you need:

*For the muffins:*

- 0.5 tsp. ground cinnamon
- 2 cups almond flour
- 0.5 cup almond milk, unsweetened
- 0.33 cup Swerve sweetener, granulated

- 3 tbsp. coconut flour
- 0.25 tsp. salt
- 3 tsp. baking powder, gluten-free
- 0.5 cup butter, unsalted
- 4 large eggs
- 0.5 tsp. vanilla extract, sugar-free
- 12 cavity muffin tin

*For the optional topping:*

- 0.5 cup almond flour
- 3 tbsp. Sukrin Gold brown sugar substitute
- 0.25 cup butter, unsalted and melted
- 2 tbsp. coconut flour
- 0.75 tsp. ground cinnamon
- saucepan

**Steps:**

1. Adjust your stove to heat at the temperature of 325° Fahrenheit.
2. Cover the 12 cavities with silicone or baking cups and set to the side.
3. Blend the salt, cinnamon, baking powder, coconut flour, Swerve, and almond flour in a glass dish until all lumpiness is no longer present.
4. Combine the vanilla extract, almond milk, eggs, and butter into the mix and blend until incorporated fully.
5. Equally distribute to the prepped cupcake tin.
6. For the optional glaze, dissolve the butter in a saucepan and turn the burner off.
7. Combine the cinnamon, coconut flour, Sukrin Gold, and almond flour in a pan and evenly distribute to the top of the batter.
8. Heat in the stove for approximately half an hour and take out to place on the countertop.
9. Wait about 10 minutes before serving and enjoy!

# Lemon Poppyseed Muffins

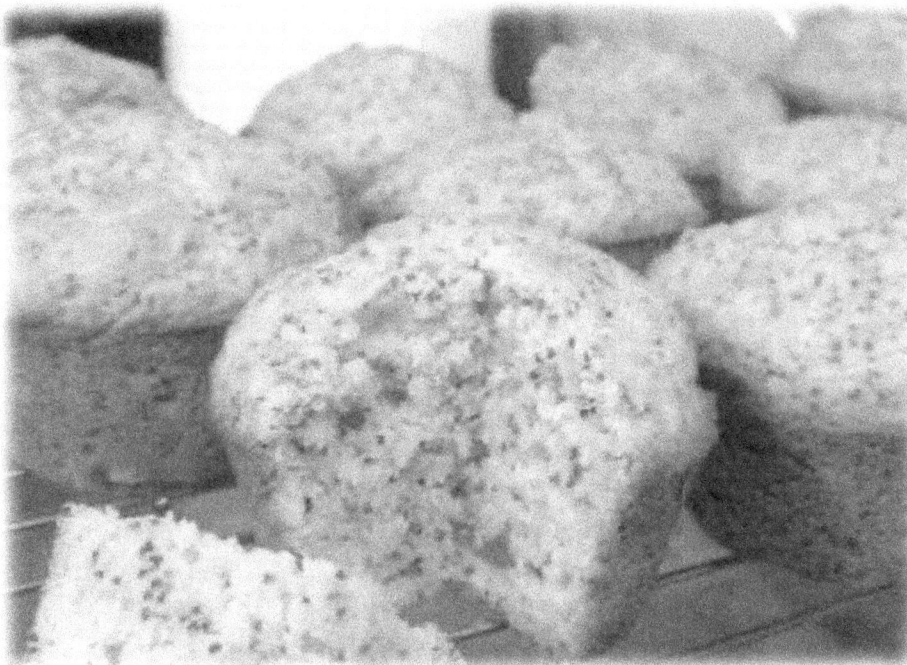

Total Prep & Cooking Time: 40 minutes
Level: Beginner
Makes: 12 Muffins
Nutritional information per muffin:
Protein: 4 grams
Net Carbs: 1.7 grams
Fat: 12 grams
Sugar: 0 grams
Calories: 130

## What you need:

- 0.25 cup golden flaxseed meal
- 0.75 cup almond flour
- 0.33 cup Erythritol sweetener, granulated
- 2 tbsp. poppy seeds
- 1 tsp. baking powder, gluten-free
- 3 large eggs
- 0.25 cup butter, salted and melted
- 2 tbsp. lemon zest
- 0.25 cup heavy cream
- 25 drops Stevia liquid

- 1 tsp. vanilla extract, sugar-free
- 3 tbsp. lemon juice
- medium saucepan
- 12 cavity muffin tin

## Steps:

1. Liquefy the butter in a saucepan and turn the burner off.
2. In the meantime, prepare a muffin tin with baking cups or silicone. Set to the side.
3. Heat your stove to the temperature of 350° Fahrenheit
4. Combine the poppy seeds, Erythritol, flaxseed meal, and almond flour with a whisk until integrated.
5. Blend the heavy cream, eggs, and melted butter until incorporated fully.
6. Finally combine the lemon juice, vanilla extract, Stevia liquid, baking powder, and lemon zest into the mix and blend well.
7. Divide the batter equally to the prepped muffin tin and heat for approximately 20 minutes.
8. Place on the countertop and wait about 10 minutes before serving.

# Loaded Chocolate Chip Muffins

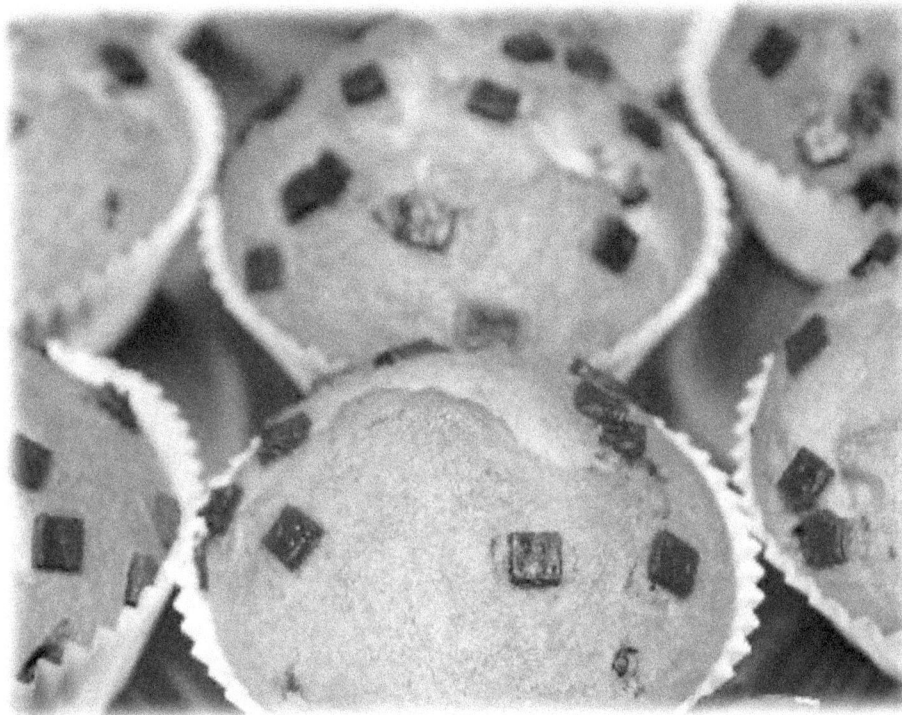

Total Prep & Cooking Time: 40 minutes
Level: Beginner
Makes: 6 Muffins
Nutritional information per muffin:
Protein: 7 grams
Net Carbs: 3 grams
Fat: 20 grams
Sugar: 0 grams
Calories: 139

## What you need:

- 1 cup almond flour
- 2 oz. butter, unsalted and melted
- 0.25 cup Erythritol sweetener, granulated
- 2 large eggs
- 1 tsp. baking powder, gluten-free
- 2 oz. almond milk, unsweetened
- 1 tsp. vanilla extract, sugar-free

- 2 oz. dark chocolate, unsweetened
- medium saucepan
- 6 cavity muffin tin

## Steps:

1. Use a saucepan to dissolve the butter completely and turn the burner off.
2. Set your stove to heat at the temperature of 355° Fahrenheit.
3. Line the cupcake tin with silicone or baking cups. Set to the side.
4. Blend the baking powder, eggs, melted butter, and almond flour in a glass dish until integrated well.
5. Combine the Erythritol, almond milk, and vanilla extract into the mix and blend completely.
6. Divide the batter evenly into the cupcake tin cavities.
7. Dice the chocolate into very thin long strips and poke them directly into the muffins.
8. Heat for the duration of 20 minutes. Wait about 10 minutes before serving warm. Enjoy!

# Strawberry Vanilla Muffins

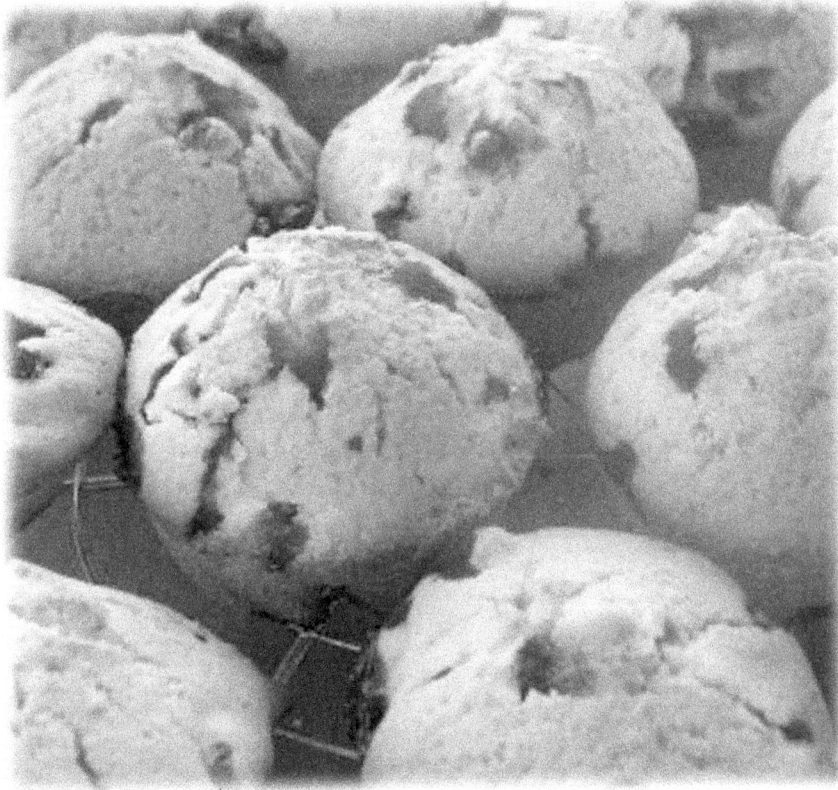

Total Prep & Cooking Time: 35 minutes
Level: Beginner
Makes: 12 Muffins
Nutritional information per muffin:
Protein: 6 grams
Net Carbs: 2.4 grams
Fat: 17 grams
Sugar: 1 gram
Calories: 122

## What you need:

- 0.25 tsp. salt
- 2 cups almond flour
- 0.5 cup butter, unsalted and melted
- 2 tsp. baking powder, gluten-free
- 0.25 cup Erythritol sweetener, granulated
- 2 tsp. vanilla extract, sugar-free
- 4 large eggs

- 0.67 cup strawberries, chopped
- 0.25 cup water
- medium saucepan
- 12 cavity muffin tin

**Steps:**

1. Use a saucepan to liquefy the butter and turn the burner off.
2. Adjust the temperature of your stove to heat at 350° Fahrenheit.
3. Cover the cavities of the cupcake tin with silicone or baking cups. Set to the side.
4. In a glass dish, blend the salt, baking powder, and almond flour, removing any lumps present.
5. Combine the vanilla extract, Erythritol, eggs, water, and butter into the dish and incorporate fully.
6. Finally, carefully integrate the strawberries.
7. Divide the batter evenly into the prepped cupcake tin and warm for approximately 18 minutes.
8. Wait about 5 minutes before enjoying.

Expert Tip:
- If you have a nut allergy, substitute coconut flour for the almond flour. Add an additional egg and 2 tbsp. of water to make the batter the correct consistency.

# Chapter 6: Cookie Recipes

## Butter Pecan Cookies

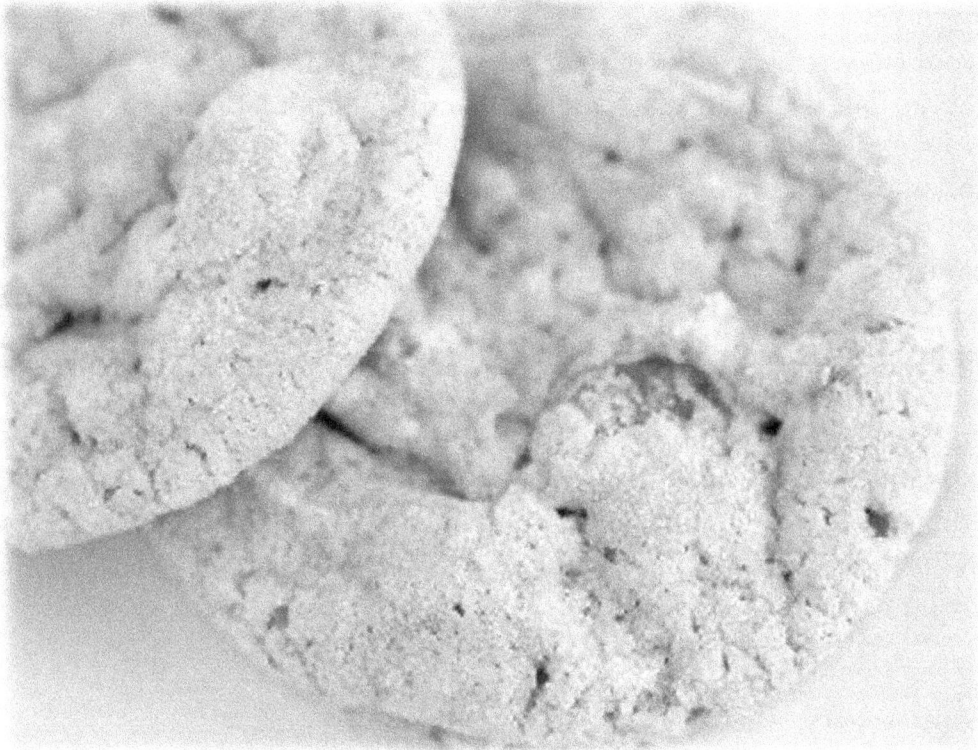

Total Prep & Cooking Time: 30 minutes
Level: Beginner
Makes: 12 Cookies
Nutritional information per cookie:
Protein: 5 grams
Net Carbs: 2.2 grams
Fat: 12 grams
Sugar: 0 grams
Calories: 240

### What you need:

- 0.33 tsp. vanilla extract, sugar-free
- 5 oz. butter, unsalted and softened
- 1 cup almond flour
- 5 oz. Swerve sweetener, granulated

- 1.25 tbsp. coconut flour
- 5 oz. toasted pecans, chopped
- 0.33 tsp. salt
- food blender or electric blender
- standard sized flat sheet with rim

## Steps:

1. Set your stove to heat at the temperature of 325° Fahrenheit.
2. Cover the flat sheet with a layer of baking lining. Set to the side.
3. Use an electric blender or a food processor to pulse the Swerve and butter for approximately 2 minutes.
4. Blend the salt, almond flour, vanilla extract, and coconut flour into the mix until integrated.
5. Carefully incorporate the chopped pecans and spoon out evenly into 12 mounds.
6. Slightly press each ball to flatten and arrange on the prepped flat pan leaving approximately 2 inches in between.
7. Heat for a total of 5 minutes and then utilize a glass with a flat-bottom to flatten the cookies to about quarter an inch thick.
8. Continue to heat for another 10 minutes and wait about 10 minutes before separating from the pan.
9. Enjoy immediately!

# Cashew Butter Cookies

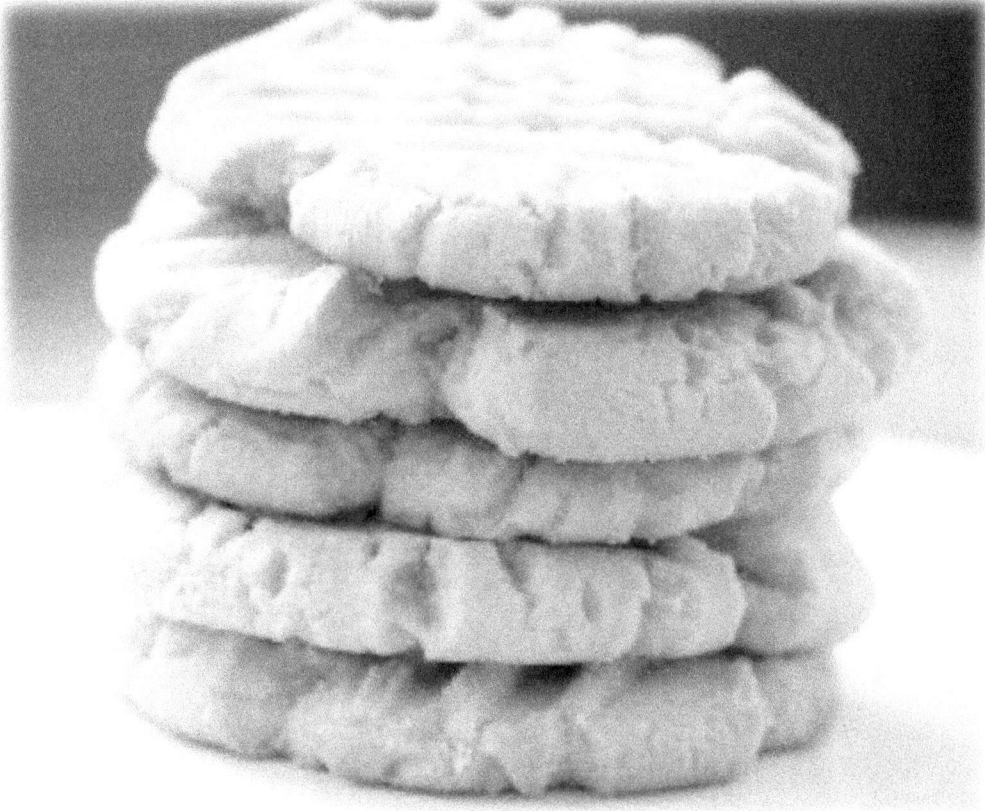

Total Prep & Cooking Time: 25 minutes
Level: Beginner
Makes: 12 Cookies
Nutritional information per cookie:
Protein: 4 grams
Net Carbs: 4.8 grams
Fat: 10 grams
Sugar: 0 grams
Calories: 116

## What you need:

- 1 large egg
- 0.5 cup Swerve sweetener, granulated
- 1 cup cashew butter
- standard sized flat sheet

## Steps:

1. Set the temperature of your stove to heat at 350° Fahrenheit.
2. Cover the flat sheet with a layer of baking lining and set aside.
3. Completely blend the egg, Swerve, and cashew butter in a glass dish until integrated fully.
4. Divide the batter evenly into 12 mounds and arrange on the prepped flat sheet with 3 inches in between.
5. Utilize a fork to apply pressure on each of the balls vertically and then horizontally.
6. Heat for approximately 12 minutes and let them sit on the countertop for 5 minutes before enjoying.

Expert Tip:

- You can also use this recipe to make peanut butter cookies by substituting the cashew butter for peanut butter.

# Oatmeal Cookies

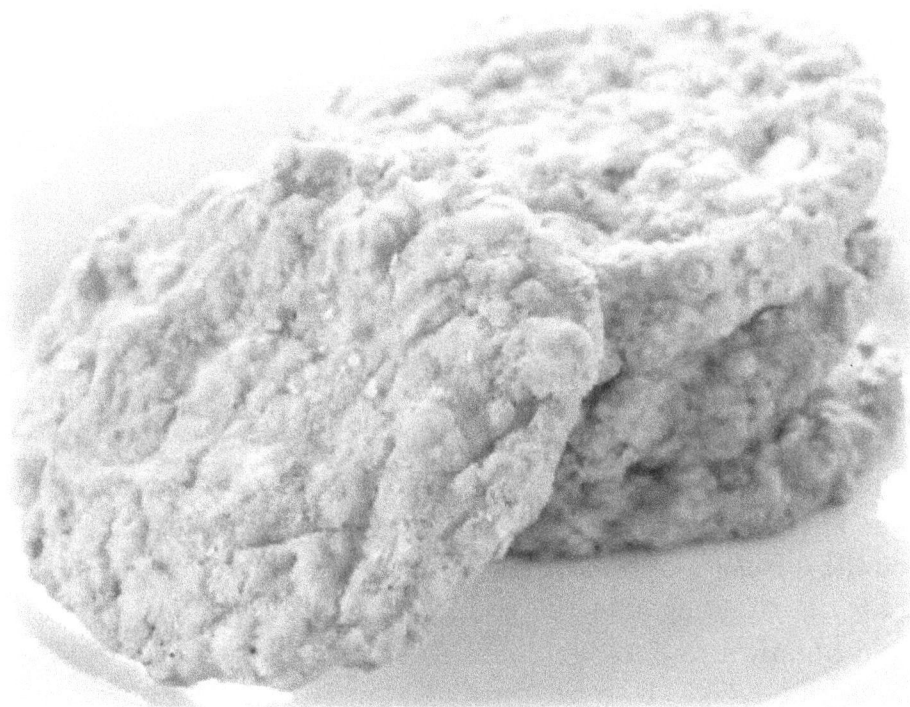

Total Prep & Cooking Time: 30 minutes
Level: Beginner
Makes: 12 Cookies
Nutritional information per cookie:
Protein: 5 grams
Net Carbs: 2.2 grams
Fat: 8 grams
Sugar: 0 grams
Calories: 240

## What you need:

- 0.33 tsp. vanilla extract
- 0.25 cup Sukrin Gold brown sugar substitute
- 0.33 cup butter, unsalted and softened
- 1.25 tbsp. oat fiber
- 0.5 tsp. ground cinnamon
- 1.25 tsp. grass-fed beef gelatin
- 0.33 tsp. baking soda
- 0.67 cup almond flour

- 0.33 tsp. salt
- 1 large egg, cold
- 1 cup almonds, sliced
- food blender
- standard sized flat sheet

## Steps:

1. Set your stove to the temperature of 350° Fahrenheit.
2. Prepare the flat sheet with a layer of baking lining and set to the side.
3. Use a food processor to pulse the vanilla extract, Sukrin Gold, and butter for approximately half a minute.
4. Blend the sliced almonds, oat fiber, cinnamon, egg, gelatin, baking soda, almond flour, and salt and pulse for another 90 seconds.
5. Spoon the batter and arrange on the prepped flat sheet leaving about 2 inches in between.
6. Heat for the duration of 8 minutes and take the sheet out of the stove.
7. Gently hit the sheet against the countertop about 5 times and continue to heat for another 6 minutes.
8. Take back out to the countertop and wait approximately 15 minutes before serving.

Expert Tips:
- If you want sweeter cookies, combine an additional 2 tbsp. of Sukrin Gold to the recipe.
- For softer cookies, reduce the sliced almonds to 1/2 cup and heat for a total of 12 minutes. The egg will need to be at room temperature if using this method.

# Raspberry Bars

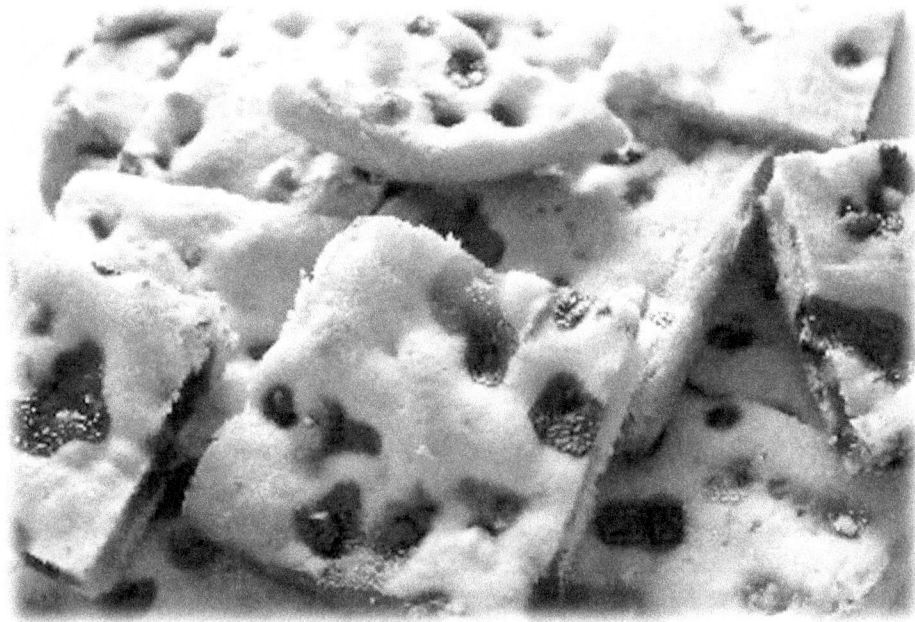

Total Prep & Cooking Time: 30 minutes
Level: Beginner
Makes: 12 Bars
Nutritional information per bar:
Protein: 3 grams
Net Carbs: 5 grams
Fat: 8 grams
Sugar: 2 grams
Calories: 72

## What you need:

- 1.5 cups almond flour
- 0.33 cup coconut flour
- 1.25 tsp. baking powder, gluten-free
- 0.67 cup Erythritol sweetener, granulated
- 1.5 tsp. vanilla extract, sugar-free
- coconut oil cooking spray
- 0.5 cup raspberries, chopped small
- 1 large egg
- 1.5 tbsp. ghee, melted
- medium saucepan
- 9 x 13 inch baking dish

## Steps:

1. Lightly coat the baking dish with coconut oil spray. Set to the side.
2. Use a saucepan to liquefy the ghee and take away from the heat.
3. Adjust the temperature of your stove to heat at 355° Fahrenheit.
4. Blend the coconut flour, Erythritol, baking powder, raspberries, and almond flour in a glass dish until incorporated.
5. Combine the vanilla extract, melted ghee, and egg until a smooth consistency.
6. Empty the batter into the prepped dish and heat for the duration of 14 minutes or until a utensil is removed from the center without residue.
7. Place on the countertop and wait about 10 minutes before slicing and serving.

Expert Tip:
- You can also create cookies with this recipe. Use a flat sheet layered with baking lining and follow steps 2 through 5. Divide the batter equally into 12 mounds and flatten by hand. Arrange on the flat sheet with 2 inches in between. Heat for a total of 12 minutes and wait about 10 minutes before serving.

# Shortbread Cookies

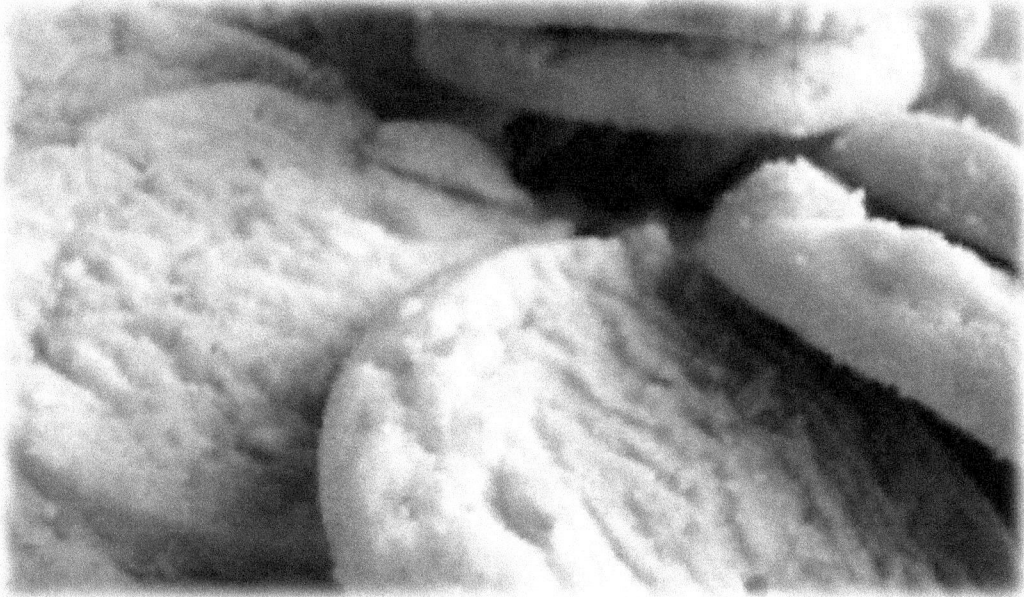

Total Prep & Cooking Time: 35 minutes
Level: Beginner
Makes: 12 Cookies
Nutritional information per cookie:
Protein: 3 grams
Net Carbs: 1 gram
Fat: 12 grams
Sugar: 0 grams
Calories: 126

## What you need:

- 1.5 cups almond flour
- 0.75 tsp. vanilla extract, sugar-free
- 0.25 cup Erythritol sweetener, granulated
- 0.125 tsp. salt
- 1 large egg
- 0.33 cup butter, unsalted and softened
- standard sized flat sheet

## Steps:

1. Heat your stove to the temperature of 300° Fahrenheit.
2. Cover a flat sheet with a layer of baking lining.

3.  Combine the vanilla extract, salt, Erythritol, and almond flour in a glass dish until incorporated.
4.  Blend the egg and butter into the mix and integrate fully.
5.  Equally section the batter into 12 mounds and apply slight pressure to flatten on the prepped flat sheet leaving approximately 2 inches in between.
6.  Heat for about 20 minutes and wait approximately 10 minutes before serving warm.

# Snickerdoodles

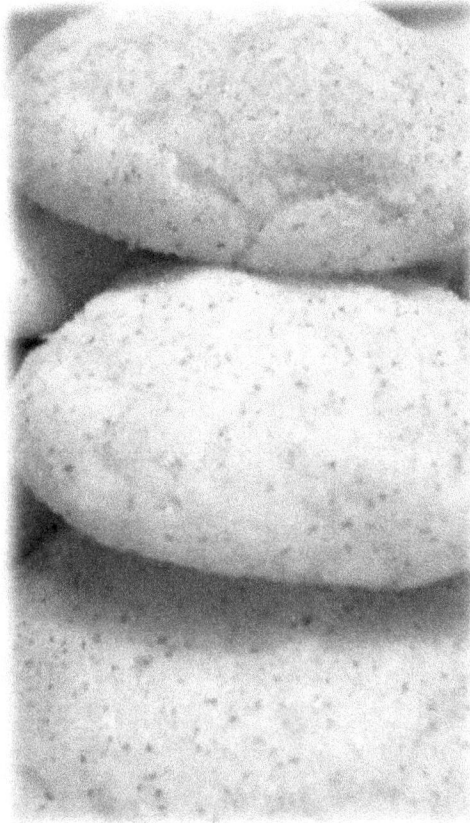

Total Prep & Cooking Time: 30 minutes
Level: Beginner
Makes: 12 Cookies
Nutritional information per cookie:
Protein: 4 grams
Net Carbs: 1.8 grams
Fat: 13 grams
Sugar: 0 grams
Calories: 139

**What you need:**

*For the dough:*

- 1.125 cup almond flour
- 0.75 tsp. vanilla extract, sugar-free
- 0.33 cup coconut flour

- 0.75 tsp. baking soda
- 1.5 tsp. ground cinnamon
- 2 large eggs
- 1.5 tsp. cream of tartar
- 0.33 tsp. xanthan gum
- 0.5 cup Swerve sweetener, granulated
- 0.125 tsp. salt
- 0.33 cup butter, unsalted
- standard sized flat sheet

*For the coating:*

- 1.5 tbsp. Swerve sweetener, granulated
- 0.75 tsp. ground cinnamon

## Steps:

1. Set your stove to heat at the temperature of 350° Fahrenheit. Layer a section of baking lining on the flat sheet and set to the side.
2. In a glass dish, blend the almond flour, salt, xanthan gum, baking soda, cream of tartar, cinnamon, and almond flour until integrated.
3. Combine the eggs, vanilla extract, Swerve, and butter into the mixture until fully incorporated.
4. To create the coating, whisk the Swerve and cinnamon in a separate dish.
5. Create 12 equal mounds and rotate in the coating before arranging on the prepped flat sheet with approximately 2 inches in between.
6. Apply slight pressure to flatten the balls and heat for 12 minutes.
7. Wait about 10 minutes before serving and enjoy!

# Sugar Cookies

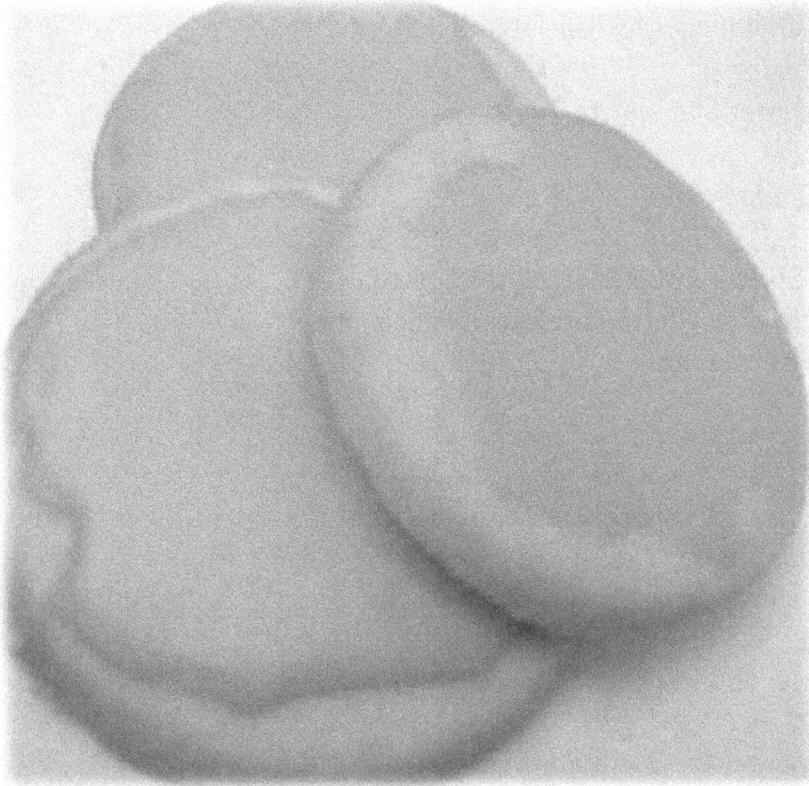

Total Prep & Cooking Time: 125 minutes / 135 minutes
Level: Intermediate/Expert
Makes: 12 Cookies
Nutritional information per cookie:
Protein: 1 gram
Net Carbs: 1 gram
Fat: 9 grams
Sugar: 0 grams
Calories: 98


## What you need:

*For the cookies:*

- 0.125 cup butter, unsalted and cubed
- 0.67 cup almond flour, blanched and sifted
- 1.5 tbsp. coconut flour, sifted
- 2 oz. Swerve sweetener, confectioner

- 1.5 tsp. salt
- 0.75 tsp. vanilla extract, sugar-free
- 1.5 tsp. almond extract, sugar-free
- 0.75 tbsp. cream cheese, full-fat and softened
- electric blender
- 2 standard sized flat sheets

*For the optional icing:*

- 0.125 cup Swerve sweetener, confectioner
- lemon juice, as needed to preferred consistency
- 0.5 tbsp. heavy cream

## Steps:

1. Use an electric blender to pulse the coconut flour, salt, Swerve, and almond flour for about half a minute.
2. Blend the butter into the mix for approximately 2 minutes until the batter is a smooth consistency.
3. Combine the almond extract, cream cheese, and vanilla extract and pulse for another minute.
4. Work the dough for about 5 minutes until it clumps together.
5. Transfer to a section of plastic wrap and completely cover the dough.
6. Refrigerate for 45 minutes.
7. Prepare the flat sheets by covering with baking lining and set to the side.
8. When the dough has set, transfer to a section of baking lining. Use an additional piece of baking lining to sandwich the dough.
9. Press to flatten with a rolling pin until approximately quarter an inch thick.
10. Transfer the dough to one flat sheet and freeze for the duration of 10 minutes.
11. After setting, use your preference in cookie cutters to section the dough into 12 shapes.
12. Use a spatula to carefully arrange the pressed cookies onto the additional prepped flat sheet leaving approximately 1 inch in between.
13. Freeze for an additional 10 minutes.
14. Adjust the temperature of your stove to heat at 325° Fahrenheit.
15. Heat the cookies for approximately 15 minutes or until the sides are turning golden.
16. Take the pan out to the countertop and wait about 15 minutes before arranging on a wire rack.
17. Wait about 10 more minutes before serving.
18. If applying the icing, in the meantime, blend the heavy cream and Swerve until the consistency is smooth. If you need to make the icing thinner, combine lemon juice

until your desired consistency.

19. After the cookies have completely cooled, apply a thin layer to each.

Expert Tips:

- If you find the batter is too watery, blend 1 tbsp. of almond flour into the mix until it reaches the desired consistency.
- You can follow steps 1 through 5 and keep the dough in the fridge for up to 2 days before following the remaining steps.
- You can freeze any leftovers up to one month. Be sure to separate each with baking lining to prevent sticking and keep in a freezer bag or lidded container.

# Thingamajigs

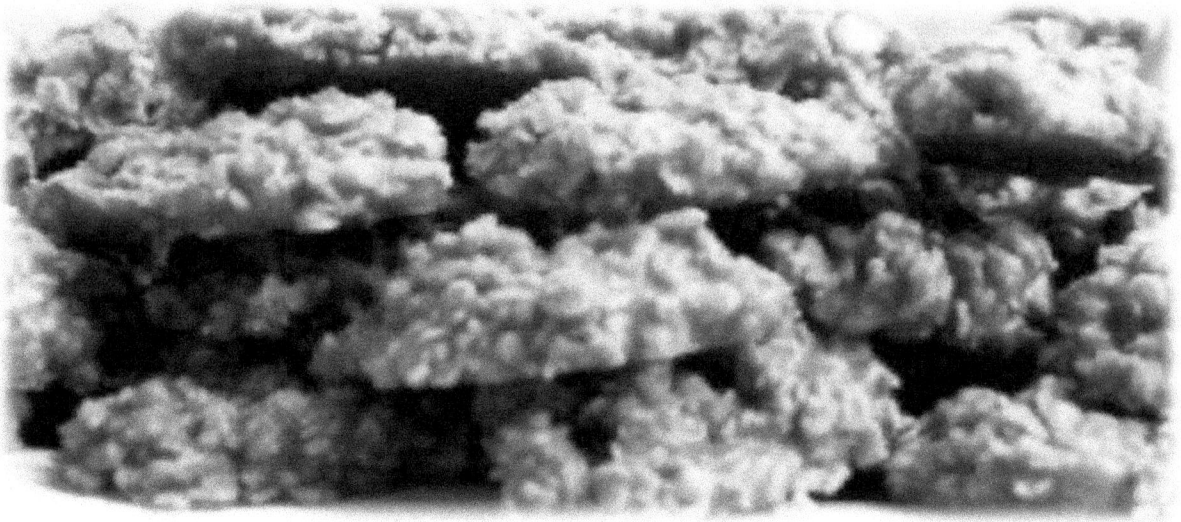

Total Prep & Cooking Time: 25 minutes
Level: Beginner
Makes: 12 Cookies, 2 cookies per helping
Nutritional information per helping:
Protein: 5 grams
Net Carbs: 3.8 grams
Fat: 16 grams
Sugar: 1 gram
Calories: 162

## What you need:

- 1.125 tbsp. butter, unsalted
- 0.67 cup coconut, unsweetened and shredded
- 0.5 cup peanut butter
- 3 drops liquid Stevia, vanilla flavour
- medium saucepan
- standard sized flat sheet

## Steps:

1. Use a saucepan to dissolve the butter completely.
2. In the meantime, layer the flat sheet with baking lining.
3. Blend the coconut, liquid Stevia, and peanut butter into the pot and integrate completely.
4. Spoon the mixture onto the prepped flat sheet leaving about 2 inches in between.

5. Freeze for the duration of 10 minutes and you serve right away. Enjoy!

Expert Tip:
- For those who are following the strict version of the Keto diet, you can substitute any nut butter instead of the peanut butter.

# Chapter 7: Pizza Crust & Breadstick Recipes

## Cauliflower Pizza Crust

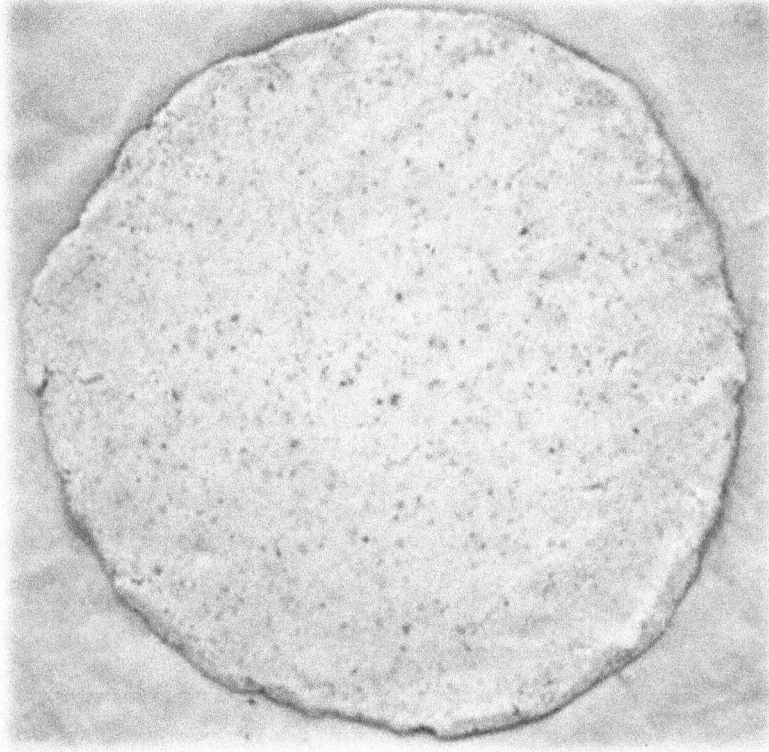

Total Prep & Cooking Time: 45 minutes
Level: Beginner
Makes: 1 Crust, 8 Slices
Nutritional information per slice:
Protein: 11 grams
Net Carbs: 5 grams
Fat: 21 grams
Sugar: 0 grams
Calories: 278

### What you need:

- 0.5 tsp. salt
- 16 oz. cauliflower florets

- 1 large egg
- 1.5 tbsp. coconut flour
- 3 tsp. avocado oil
- 0.5 tsp. Italian seasoning
- 1 tsp. coconut oil
- food blender
- large skillet
- large flat sheet or pizza pan

## Steps:

1. Set your oven to heat at the temperature of 405° Fahrenheit.
2. Pulse the cauliflower in a food blender for approximately 60 seconds until it is a crumbly consistency.
3. Heat the coconut oil and cauliflower in a frypan for approximately 5 minutes as it becomes tender.
4. Transfer the cauliflower to a kitchen towel and twist to eliminate the extra water. Repeat this step as many times as necessary to make sure the moisture has been eliminated.
5. Prepare your pizza pan or flat sheet with a section of baking lining and set to the side.
6. In a glass dish, blend the riced cauliflower, salt, egg, coconut flour, avocado oil, and Italian seasoning and integrate until it thickens.
7. Flatten the dough onto the prepped pan to no less than a quarter inch.
8. Heat for 25 minutes if then and up to half an hour if thicker.
9. Complete with your favorite toppings and finish in the stove for another 5 minutes. Enjoy!

Expert Tip:
- For the toppings, be creative with vegetable and meat combinations. The first layer should be your sauce and then layer the meat and vegetables and top with cheese to ensure all ingredients heat properly.

# Cauliflower Breadsticks

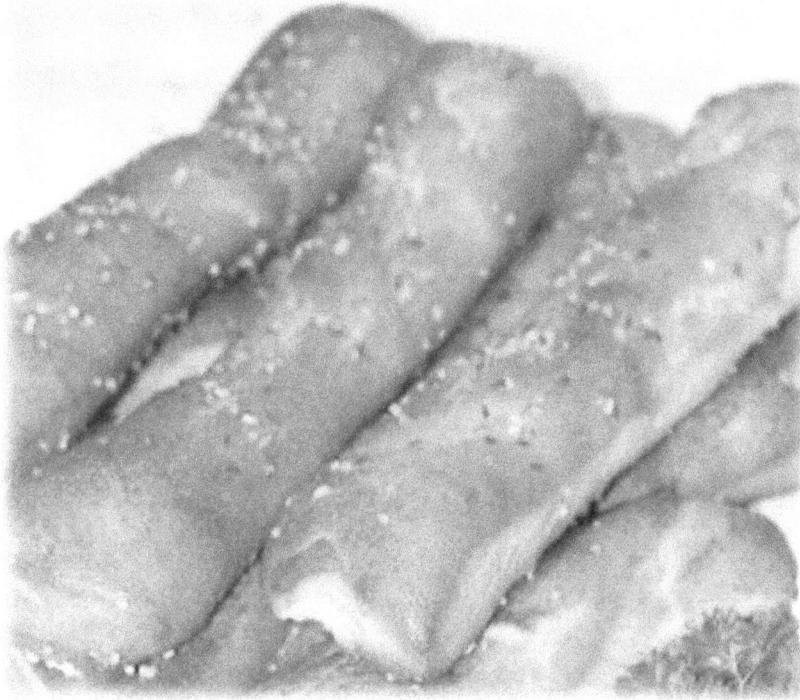

Total Prep & Cooking Time: 45 minutes
Level: Beginner
Makes: 8 Breadsticks, 2 breadsticks per helping
Nutritional information per helping:
Protein: 13 grams
Net Carbs: 4 grams
Fat: 10 grams
Sugar: 1 gram
Calories: 165

## What you need:

- 0.5 tsp. ground pepper
- 2 cups riced cauliflower
- 0.5 tsp. garlic powder
- 1 tsp. Italian seasoning
- 0.25 cup grated Parmesan cheese
- 2 large eggs
- 0.5 tsp. salt
- 1 cup Mexican cheese blend, shredded

- 2 tbsp. coconut oil
- food blender
- large skillet
- 9 x 3 inch glass baking pan or standard sized flat sheet with rim

## Steps:

1. Layer a section of baking lining on your desired pan. Set to the side.
2. Crumble the cauliflower in a food blender for approximately 60 seconds.
3. Heat the cauliflower and coconut oil in a frypan for approximately 5 minutes as it becomes soft.
4. Distribute the cauliflower to a kitchen towel and wring to eliminate the extra moisture. Repeat this step as many times as necessary to make sure the moisture has been removed.
5. Adjust the heat of your stove to the temperature of 350° Fahrenheit.
6. Pulse the eggs, riced cauliflower, Mexican cheese blend, salt, Italian seasoning, garlic, and pepper for approximately 2 minutes.
7. Distribute to the prepped pan and apply slight pressure to evenly spread throughout.
8. For half an hour, heat in the stove and move to the countertop.
9. Dust with the parmesan cheese and set the stove to broil.
10. Warm for approximately 3 minutes and put back onto the countertop.
11. Section into 8 even pieces and serve immediately.

# Crunchy Cheese Sticks

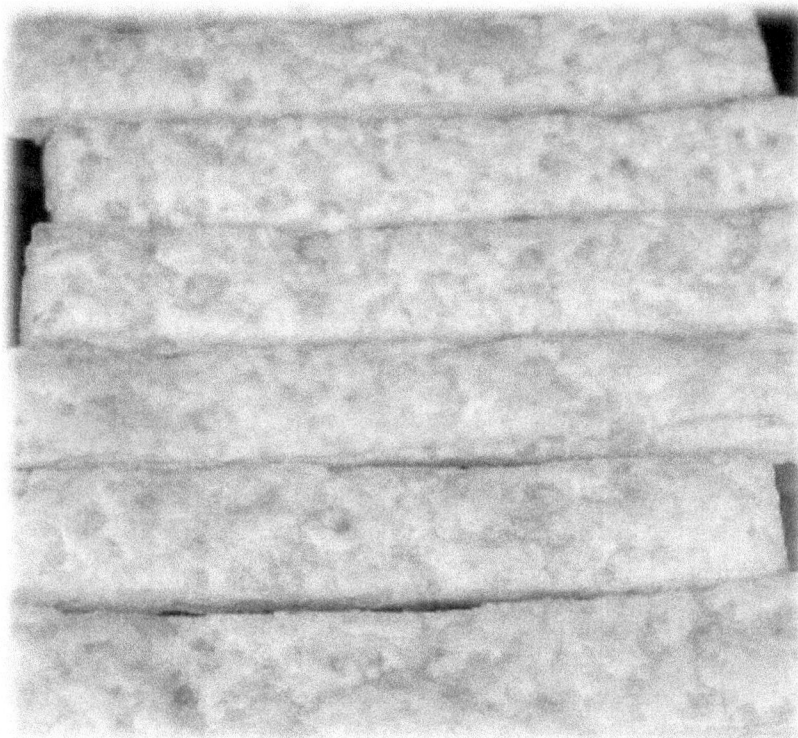

Total Prep & Cooking Time: 30 minutes
Level: Beginner
Makes: 8 Breadsticks
Nutritional information per breadstick:
Protein: 17 grams
Net Carbs: 3 grams
Fat: 23 grams
Sugar: 1 gram
Calories: 299


**What you need:**

*For the breadsticks:*

- 1.33 cup mozzarella cheese, shredded
- 4.5 tbsp. butter, unsalted, melted and cooled
- 0.33 cup coconut flour
- 1 oz. cream cheese, full-fat and softened
- 0.5 cup parmesan cheese, shredded

- 4 large eggs
- 0.25 tsp. salt
- 1 tsp. Italian seasoning
- 0.5 tsp. garlic powder
- 0.25 tsp. baking powder, gluten-free
- medium saucepan
- 11 x 7 inch glass baking dish

*For the topping:*

- 2 cups mozzarella cheese shredded
- 0.5 tsp Italian seasoning
- 0.25 cup parmesan cheese shredded

## Steps:

1. Dissolve the butter completely in the saucepan and turn the burner off.
2. Set your stove to heat at the temperature of 400° Fahrenheit.
3. Spray the coconut oil onto the baking dish and set to the side.
4. Blend the cream cheese, salt, eggs, and melted butter until smooth.
5. Combine the garlic powder, Italian seasoning, baking powder, and coconut flour into the mix until integrated fully.
6. Finally, blend the parmesan and mozzarella cheese into the batter.
7. Distribute into the prepped pan and press with a spatula to ensure it is even throughout.
8. Dust the toppings of mozzarella cheese, Italian seasoning, and parmesan cheese on the batter.
9. Heat for 8 minutes and remove to the stove top. Divide into 8 sections with a pizza cutter. Continue to heat for an additional 7 minutes.
10. Turn the stove to the setting of broil and complete the process by heating for 2 more minutes.
11. Serve immediately and enjoy!

# Italian Breadsticks

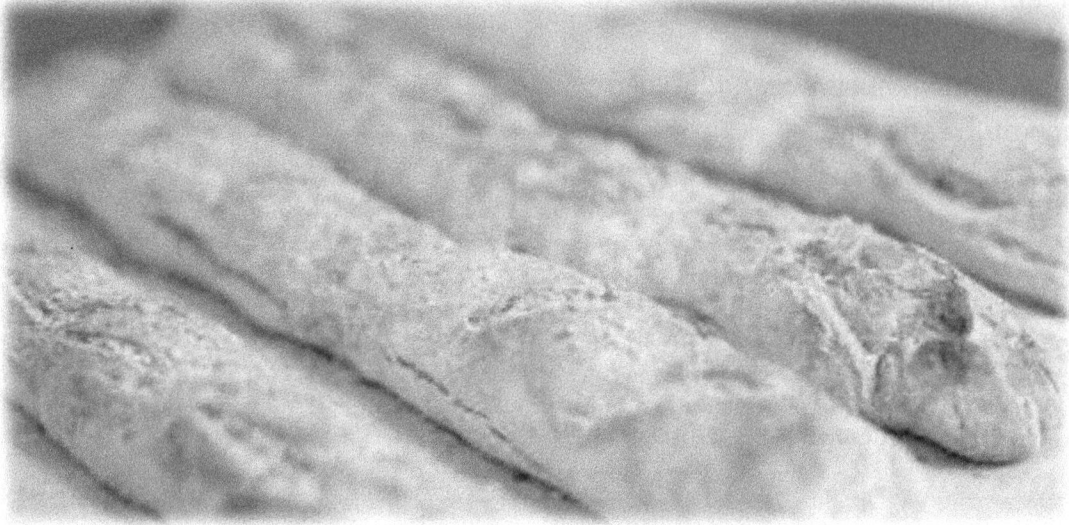

Total Prep & Cooking Time: 25 minutes
Level: Beginner
Makes: 8 Breadsticks
Nutritional information per breadstick:
Protein: 8 grams
Net Carbs: 2 grams
Fat: 10 grams
Sugar: 0 grams
Calories: 130

## What you need:

- 1 tsp. baking powder, gluten-free
- 1.5 oz. cream cheese, full-fat
- 6 oz. almond flour
- 0.5 tbsp. nutritional yeast
- 1 clove garlic, grated
- 0.25 tsp. basil seasoning
- 10 oz. mozzarella cheese, shredded and part-skim milk
- 0.5 tsp. garlic salt
- 1 large eggs
- 3 tsp. parmesan cheese, grated
- 0.5 tbsp. psyllium husk powder
- 4 tbsp. olive oil, separated

- 1 tsp. parsley seasoning
- standard sized flat sheet

## Steps:

1. Adjust the temperature on your stove to heat at 400° Fahrenheit.
2. Cover the flat sheet with a layer of baking lining and set to the side.
3. In a glass dish, blend the baking powder, garlic salt, parsley, oregano, basil, nutritional yeast, psyllium husk powder, and almond flour with a whisk to ensure no lumps are present.
4. Use a microwave safe dish to nuke the cream cheese and mozzarella for 60 seconds. Toss and then heat again for half a minute.
5. Combine the melted cheese and garlic into the mix.
6. Use up to 2 tbsp. of olive oil to grease your hands.
7. Section the dough into 8 equal pieces and roll into long sections.
8. Arrange the sticks on the prepped sheet and heat for the duration of 12 minutes.
9. Brush the leftover 2 tbsp. of olive oil over the sticks and continue to heat for another 3 minutes.
10. Serve while hot and enjoy!

# Mozzarella Pizza Crust

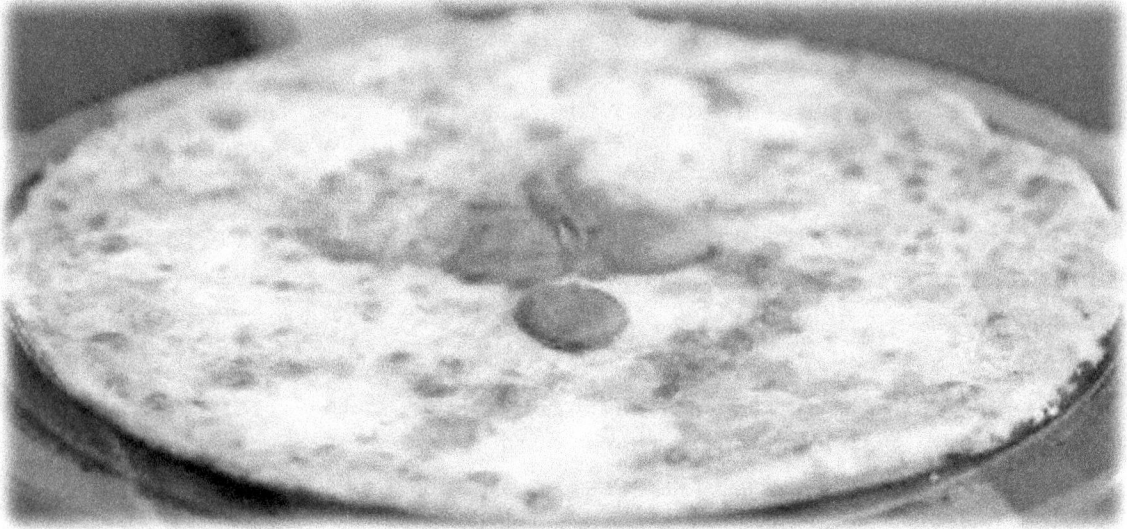

Total Prep & Cooking Time: 30 minutes
Level: Beginner
Makes: 1 Crust, 8 Slices
Nutritional information per slice:
Protein: 10 grams
Net Carbs: 1.4 grams
Fat: 6 grams
Sugar: 2 grams
Calories: 190

## What you need:

- 1.5 cups mozzarella cheese, shredded
- 0.75 cup almond flour
- 1 whole egg
- 2 tbsp. cream cheese, full-fat
- 0.25 tsp. salt
- pizza pan or large flat sheet

## Steps:

1. Set your stove to heat at the temperature of 350° Fahrenheit.
2. Use a microwave-safe dish to nuke the almond flour, mozzarella, and cream cheese for approximately 60 seconds until liquefied.

3. Toss the cheese and heat for an additional half minute.
4. Blend the salt and egg into the cheese for about half a minute.
5. Place a section of baking lining on the counter and transfer the dough to the middle. Use another section of baking lining to place on top.
6. Flatten to no less than a quarter of an inch. Separate the top baking lining and transfer to the pan of choice.
7. Heat for approximately 13 minutes until turning golden.
8. Layer with your toppings of choice and heat for about 5 minutes.
9. Serve hot and enjoy!

Expert Tip:

- If you have a nut allergy, you can substitute the almond flour with 1/4 cup of coconut flour.

# Savory Garlic Breadsticks

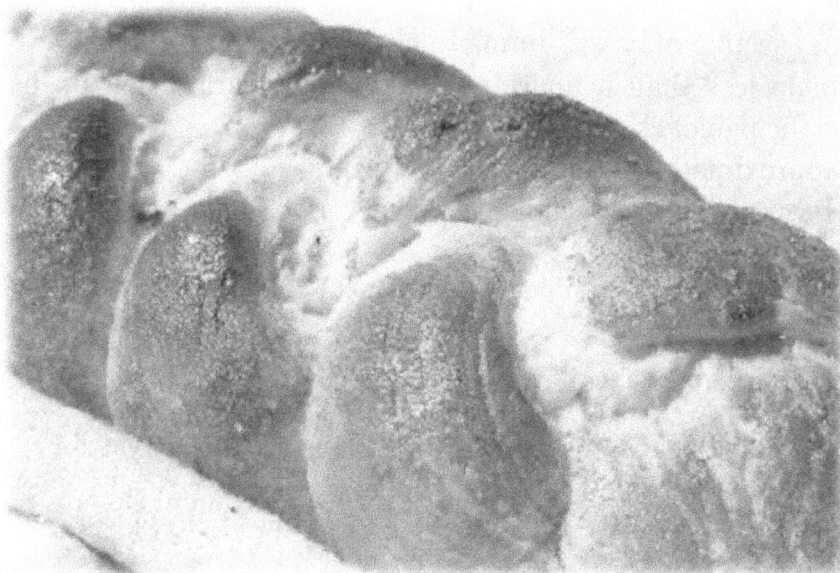

Total Prep & Cooking Time: 25 minutes
Level: Intermediate/Expert
Makes: 8 Breadsticks
Nutritional information per breadstick:
Protein: 9 grams
Net Carbs: 2.1 grams
Fat: 18 grams
Sugar: 1 gram
Calories: 210

## What you need:

*For the topping:*

- 2 tbsp. butter, unsalted and melted
- 0.25 tsp. salt
- 2 cloves of garlic, crushed

*For the dough:*

- 0.33 cup coconut flour
- 8 oz. mozzarella cheese, shredded
- 0.33 cup almond flour

- 2 oz. cream cheese, full-fat
- 0.33 cup golden flax seed, ground
- 1 large egg
- standard sized flat sheet
- food blender
- medium saucepan

## Steps:

1. Set your stove to the temperature of 400° Fahrenheit.
2. Cover the flat pan with a layer of baking lining. Set to the side.
3. Combine the topping ingredients of butter and garlic to the saucepan and heat for approximately 3 minutes. Turn the burner off and leave to the side.
4. Nuke the mozzarella cheese in a microwave-safe dish for 60 seconds. Gently toss and heat again for 30 seconds.
5. Pulse the coconut flour, cream cheese, golden flax seed, egg, and almond flour into the melted cheese in a food blender until it becomes a thick consistency after approximately 3 minutes.
6. Transfer to a section of baking lining and sandwich with another piece of baking lining.
7. Flatten in a rectangle to approximately half an inch. Section into 8 equal strips. Divide each strip into 3 sections.
8. Dampen your hands as much as needed for the next four steps.
9. Arrange 3 of the strips side by side and press them together at the top.
10. Create a braid pattern by alternating the right strip over the middle strip and then the left strip over the middle strip until all the dough is braided.
11. Press the base of the dough to complete the braid. Transfer to the prepped sheet.
12. Repeat steps 7 through 9 for all the breadsticks.
13. Apply a coat of the garlic butter and dust with salt.
14. Heat for the duration of 15 minutes. Apply the leftover garlic butter and heat for an additional 10 minutes.
15. Serve immediately and enjoy!

# Zucchini Pizza Crust

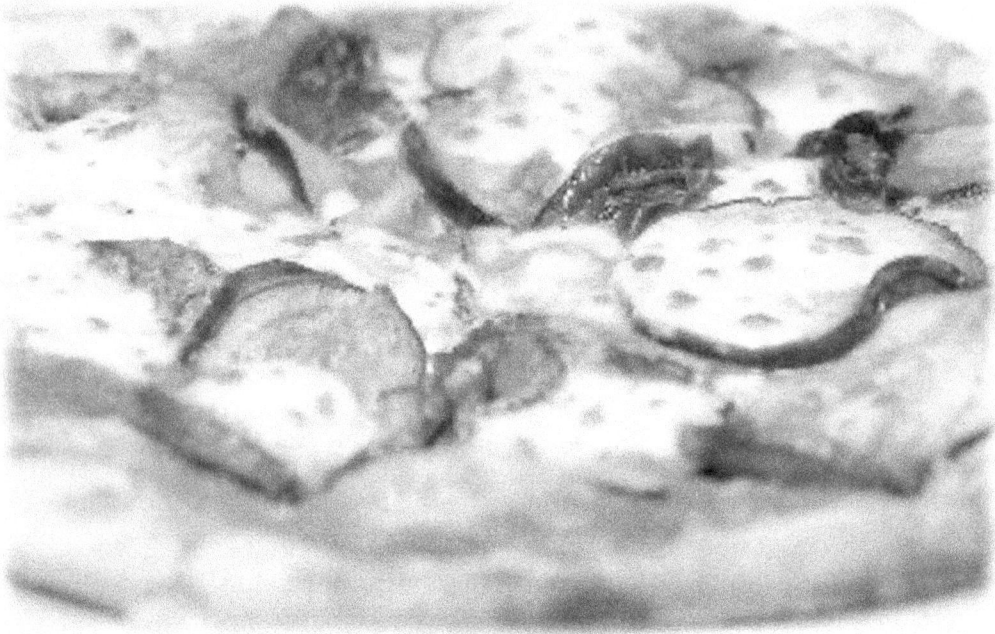

Total Prep & Cooking Time: 60 minutes
Level: Beginner
Makes: 1 Crust, 8 Slices
Nutritional information per slice:
Protein: 7 grams
Net Carbs: 4 grams
Fat: 8 grams
Sugar: 1 gram
Calories: 127

## What you need:

- 4 cups zucchini, shredded
- 1 cup almond flour
- 2.75 tbsp. coconut flour
- 4 tbsp. nutritional yeast
- 1.33 tbsp. Italian seasoning
- 0.75 tsp. salt
- 3 large eggs
- kitchen grater
- large flat sheet or pizza pan

## Steps:

1. Adjust the temperature of your stove to heat at 400° Fahrenheit.
2. Cover the desired pan with a layer of baking lining and set to the side.
3. Use a kitchen grater to shred the zucchini using the largest holes available.
4. Transfer to a kitchen towel and wring to release all excess moisture.
5. In a glass dish, blend the coconut flour, zucchini, salt, Italian seasoning, nutritional yeast, eggs, and almond flour until integrated and thickened.
6. Distribute to the prepped sheet and flatten to no less than quarter an inch by hand.
7. Heat for the duration of 20 minutes. Turn the crust over and warm for another 10 minutes.
8. Layer with your preferred toppings and heat for another 13 minutes.
9. Wait about 10 minutes before slicing and serving. Enjoy!

# Chapter 8: Bagel Recipes

## Bacon Bagels

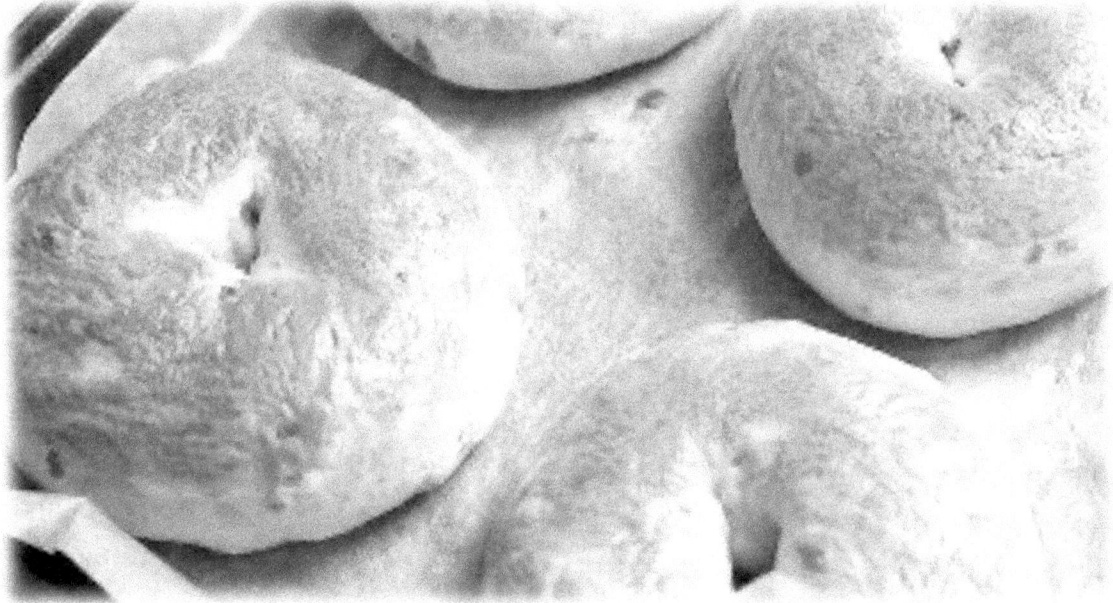

Total Prep & Cooking Time: 25 minutes
Level: Beginner/Intermediate
Makes: 6 Bagels
Nutritional information per bagel:
Protein: 11 grams
Net Carbs: 2.3 grams
Fat: 13 grams
Sugar: 1 gram
Calories: 173

**What you need:**

- 2 large eggs, beaten
- 1.5 cup almond flour
- 0.75 tbsp. baking powder, gluten-free
- 0.33 tsp. salt
- 2 cups mozzarella cheese, shredded
- 1.5 oz. cream cheese, full-fat
- 4 strips bacon, uncooked and chopped

- large skillet
- standard sized flat sheet

## Steps:

1. Heat the chopped bacon in a frypan for approximately 5 minutes or until your desired crispiness and take away from the burner.
2. Use a spoon with slots to transfer the bacon to a kitchen paper covered plate. Leave to the side.
3. Set your stove to heat at the temperature of 400° Fahrenheit.
4. Prepare the flat sheet by covering with a section of the baking lining. Set aside.
5. In a microwave-safe dish, nuke the cream cheese and mozzarella for 2 minutes while tossing approximately even half minute.
6. Blend the salt, baking powder and almond flour, eggs, and bacon with the cheese. Wet your hands and work by hand until the batter thickens.
7. Section into 8 equal portions and roll into a log.
8. Pinch the ends together to create a circle and arrange on the prepped flat sheet.
9. For approximately 12 minutes, heat the bagels until golden.
10. Serve while hot. Enjoy!

# Blueberry Bagels

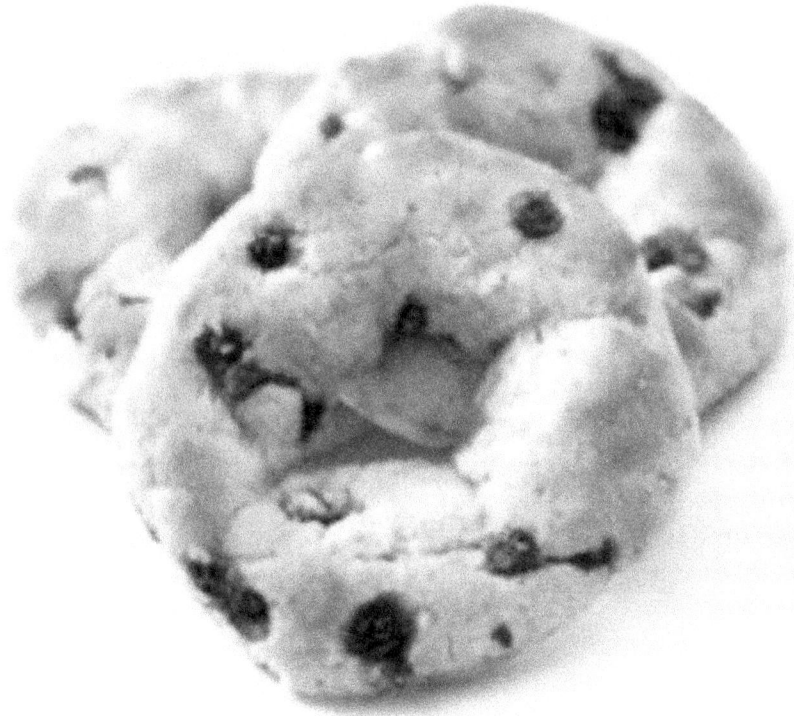

Total Prep & Cooking Time: 120 minutes
Level: Intermediate/Expert
Makes: 8 Bagels
Nutritional information per bagel:
Protein: 6 grams
Net Carbs: 3.5 grams
Fat: 15 grams
Sugar: 1 gram
Calories: 197

## What you need:

- 0.33 tsp. salt
- 0.75 tbsp. active dry yeast
- 1.5 tsp. honey (See Expert Tips Below)
- 0.125 cup olive oil
- 2 tbsp. whey protein isolate
- 0.33 cup lukewarm water

- 0.75 tbsp. Sukrin Gold brown sugar substitute
- 1.125 cup almond flour
- 0.75 tbsp. apple cider vinegar
- 0.25 cup golden flaxseed meal
- 0.75 cup blueberries
- 1.5 tsp. baking powder, gluten-free
- 0.33 tsp. ground cinnamon
- 1.75 tsp. xanthan gum
- 1 large egg
- 1.5 egg whites
- medium saucepan
- electric blender
- standard sized flat sheet

## Steps:

1. Cover the flat sheet with a section of baking lining and set to the side.
2. Combine the maple syrup and yeast in a glass dish.
3. Warm the water to the temperature of 105° Fahrenheit in the saucepan and blend with the yeast.
4. Use a kitchen towel to place over the dish and set to the side for 7 minutes. If the mixture does not bubble, you need to repeat steps 1 through 3 again.
5. Meanwhile in a separate glass dish, blend the almond flour, salt, cinnamon, baking powder, xanthan gum, Erythritol, whey protein isolate, and psyllium husk until integrated.
6. In the yeast dish, combine the egg, vinegar, olive oil, and egg whites. Use an electric blender to whip for approximately 2 minutes.
7. Slowly pulse the flour mix into the batter over the matter of 2 additional minutes.
8. Finely blend the blueberries into the mix.
9. Douse your hands with water and section the dough into 8 equal mounds.
10. Use your finger to poke a hole into the middle of each and form the donut shape for each mound.
11. Arrange on the prepped flat sheet and apply a coat of olive oil to each.
12. Cover with a layer of plastic wrap and then a kitchen towel. Set on top of the stove for approximately 40 minutes.
13. About 20 minutes after, set your stove to heat at the temperature of 350° Fahrenheit.
14. Once the bagels have risen properly, heat for approximately 23 minutes or until golden.
15. Wait at least 15 minutes before serving and enjoy!

Expert Tips:

- Do not worry about the maple syrup not being part of the Keto diet. It is simply to activate the yeast and all the sugar will be burned off during the cooking process.
- These bagels will keep on the counter up to 2 days when stored in a lidded tub. They will also stay fresh for up to 2 weeks in the freezer.
- Feel free to substitute more psyllium husk in place of the golden flaxseed meal.
- If you do not have xanthan gum, replace it with 1.5 tbsp. of ground flax seeds that have been ground down to powder in a food blender.

# Buttery Bagels

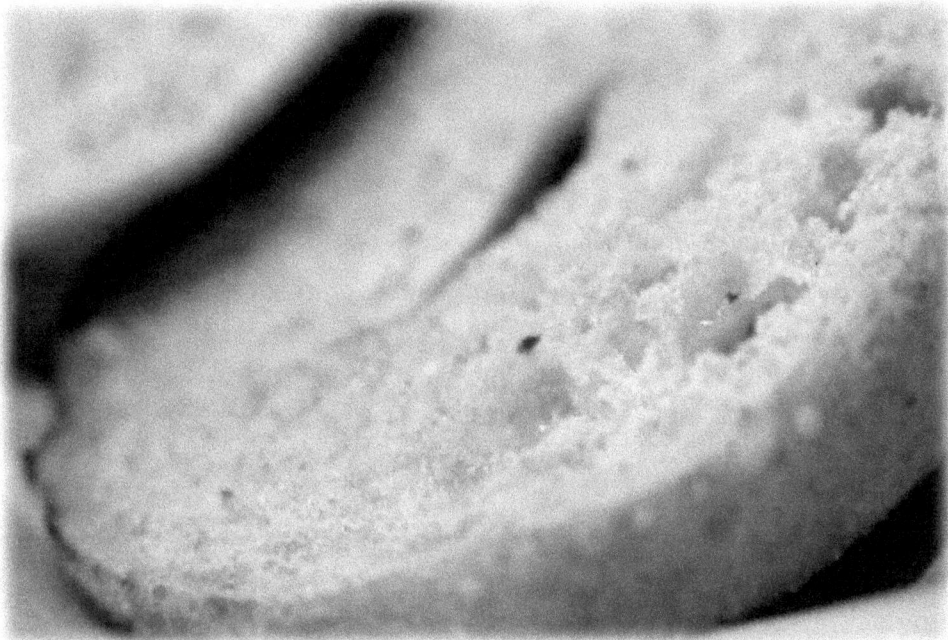

Total Prep & Cooking Time: 40 minutes
Level: Beginner
Makes: 6 Bagels
Nutritional information per bagel:
Protein: 6 grams
Carbs: 1.2 grams
Fat: 3 grams
Sugar: 1 gram
Calories: 83

## What you need:

- 0.5 tsp. baking soda
- 1.75 tbsp. butter, unsalted and melted
- 3 large eggs, separated
- 0.25 tsp. cream of tartar
- 2 tbsp. coconut flour, sifted
- 0.25 tsp. cream of tartar
- 1.75 tbsp. cream cheese, full-fat and softened
- 2 tsp. Swerve sweetener, granulated
- 0.125 tsp. salt.
- coconut oil cooking spray

- medium saucepan
- 6 cavity donut pan

**Steps:**

1. Use a saucepan to liquefy the butter completely and turn the burner off.
2. Set your stove to the temperature of 300° Fahrenheit.
3. Liberally coat the pan with the coconut oil spray and set to the side.
4. Set out 2 glass dishes and divide the eggs between whites and yolks.
5. Blend the cream of tartar with the egg whites and pulse with an electric blender for the duration of approximately 5 minutes.
6. Combine the egg yolks with the salt, baking soda, Swerve, coconut flour, melted butter, and cream cheese.
7. Gently blend the whipped eggs into the mix and be sure not to blend completely.
8. Equally distribute the batter to the prepped pan. Be sure there is no excess dripped onto the pan.
9. Heat for approximately 23 minutes and transfer to the countertop.
10. Separate the bagel from the pan by using a knife and serve after about 5 minutes. Enjoy!

# Cheese Bagels

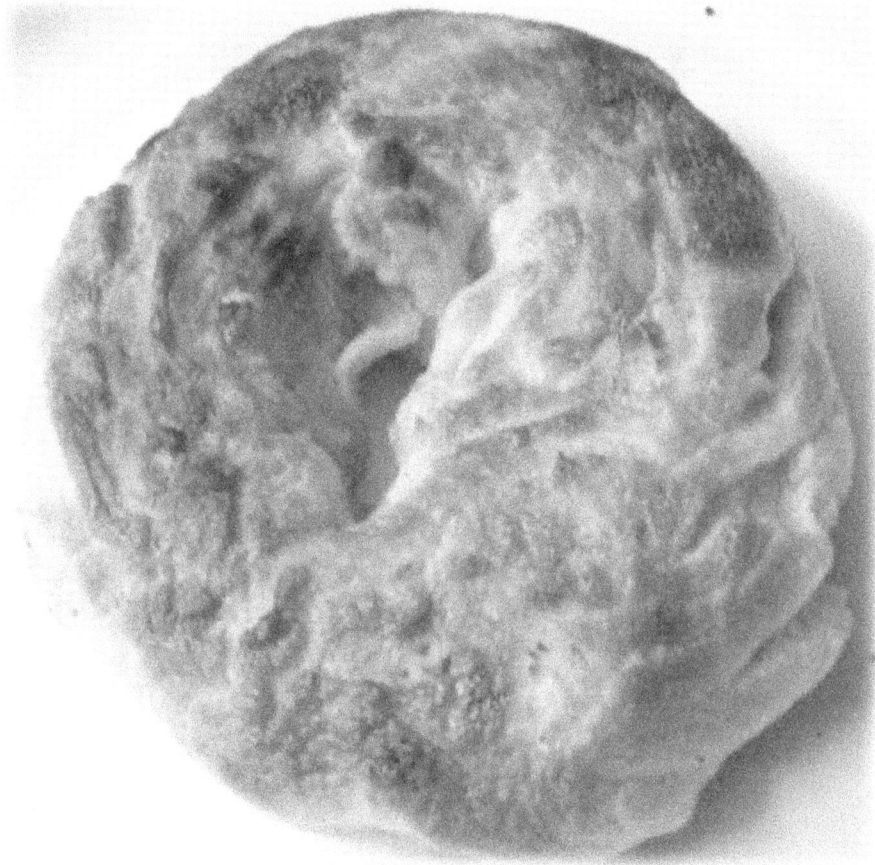

Total Prep & Cooking Time: 30 minutes
Level: Beginner
Makes: 6 Bagels
Nutritional information per bagel:
Protein: 12 grams
Carbs: 2.5 grams
Fat: 16 grams
Sugar: 0 grams
Calories: 203

## What you need:

- 1.5 cups mozzarella cheese, shredded
- 0.75 tbsp. baking powder, gluten-free
- 0.25 cup cream cheese, full-fat
- 2 large eggs
- 1.25 cup almond flour

- 0.75 cup Asiago cheese, shredded and separated
- 0.33 tsp. salt
- standard sized flat sheet

## Steps:

1. Adjust the heat of your stove to the temperature of 400° Fahrenheit.
2. Prepare the sheet with a layer of baking lining and set to the side.
3. Blend the salt, baking powder, eggs, and almond flour in a glass dish until all lumpiness is not present.
4. Nuke the cream cheese and mozzarella in a microwave-safe dish for one minute. Toss and then heat for another half minute.
5. Blend the melted cheese into the flour mix along with 1/2 cup of the Asiago cheese until it thickens.
6. Divide the dough into 8 sections of equal measure and create mounds out of each.
7. Use your fingers to press holes into the middle of each and arrange on the prepped sheet.
8. Dust with the leftover 1/4 cup of Asiago cheese and heat for the duration of 20 minutes.
9. Serve immediately and enjoy!

# Rosemary Bagels

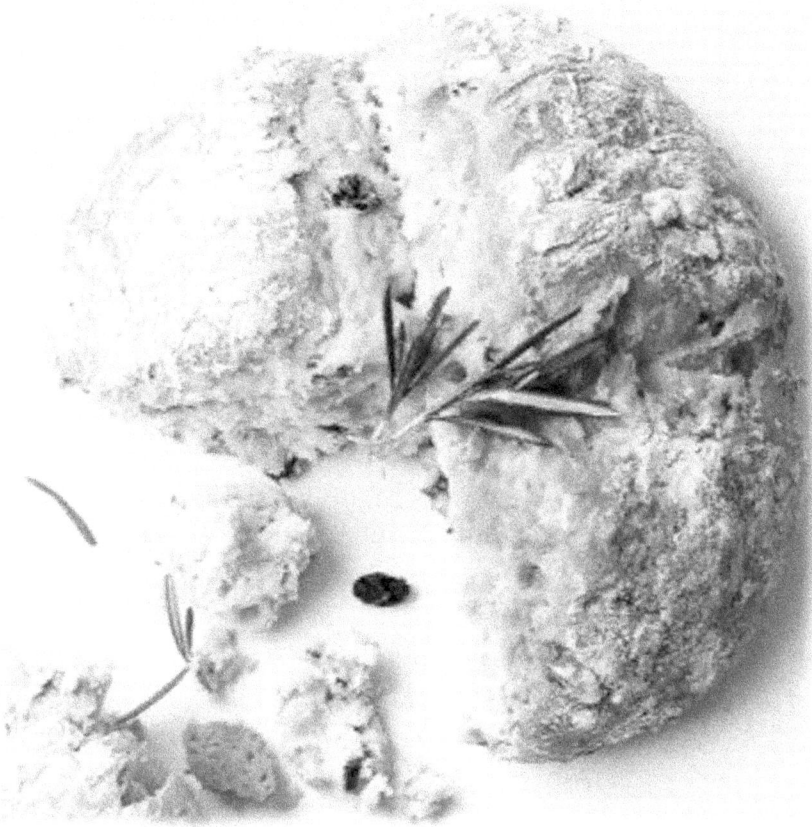

Total Prep & Cooking Time: 70 minutes
Level: Beginner
Makes: 6 Bagels
Nutritional information per bagel:
Protein: 13 grams
Carbs: 4.5 grams
Fat: 23 grams
Sugar: 1 gram
Calories: 285

## What you need:

- 1.125 tsp. baking soda
- 4.5 tbsp. psyllium husk powder
- 1.125 tsp. xanthan gum
- 2 large egg

- 0.33 tsp. salt
- 4.5 egg whites
- 0.75 cup warm water
- 1.5 tbsp. rosemary, chopped
- 2.5 cups almond flour
- avocado oil cooking spray
- food blender
- 6 cavity donut pan

## Steps:

1. Set the temperature of your stove to heat at 250° Fahrenheit.
2. Use a food blender to pulse the salt, baking soda, xanthan gum, and almond flour for about half a minute.
3. Combine the warm water and eggs and pulse for another half minute.
4. Blend the psyllium husk in the blender for another 30 seconds.
5. Apply the avocado oil spray to the donut tray and distribute the batter evenly into each cavity.
6. Dust evenly with rosemary and heat for a total of 45 minutes.
7. Wait for 15 minutes before serving and enjoy!

# Conclusion

Thank you again for purchasing your copy of the *"Keto Bread Cookbook"*.
I hope that you found the recipes easy to follow and enjoyable to create in your kitchen.

Now that you know that you can still enjoy wonderful tasting breads on the keto diet, my wish is that you get creative with the recipes and use them as a base to experiment with other delicious varieties now and in the future.

Knowing that these recipes will couple well with the other Keto recipes, this will add even more diversity to the meals that you can enjoy while focusing on your personal weight loss goals.

I will you continued success on your Keto journey, and happy baking!

# Other books by Serena Baker

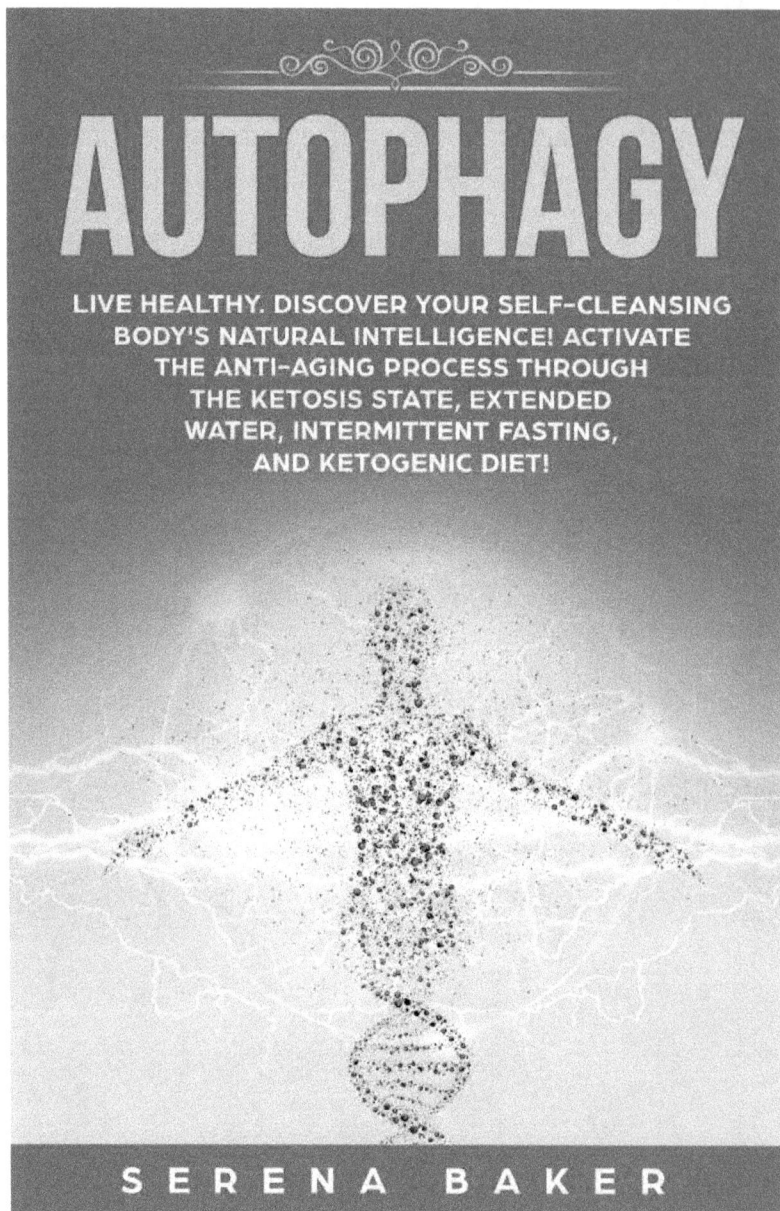

## Autophagy

*Discover your self-cleansing body's natural intelligence!*

# INTERMITTENT FASTING
## *for Women*

LEARN HOW YOU CAN USE THIS SCIENCE TO SUPPORT YOUR HORMONES, LOSE WEIGHT, ENJOY YOUR FOOD, AND LIVE A HEALTHY LIFE WITHOUT SUFFERING FROM YOUR DIETARY HABITS

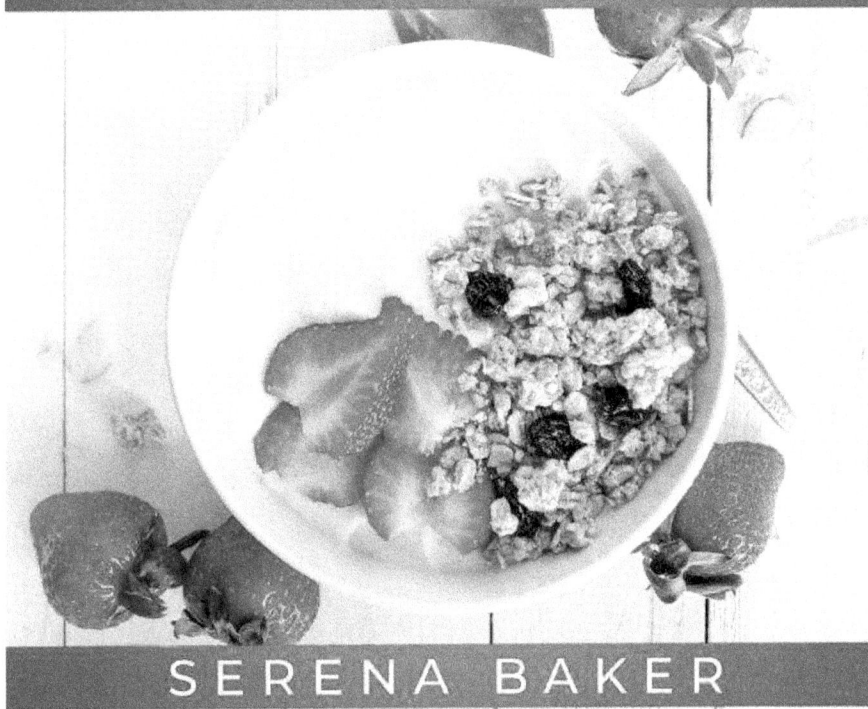

## SERENA BAKER

# *Intermittent Fasting for Women*

*Intermittent Fasting designed specifically for Women*

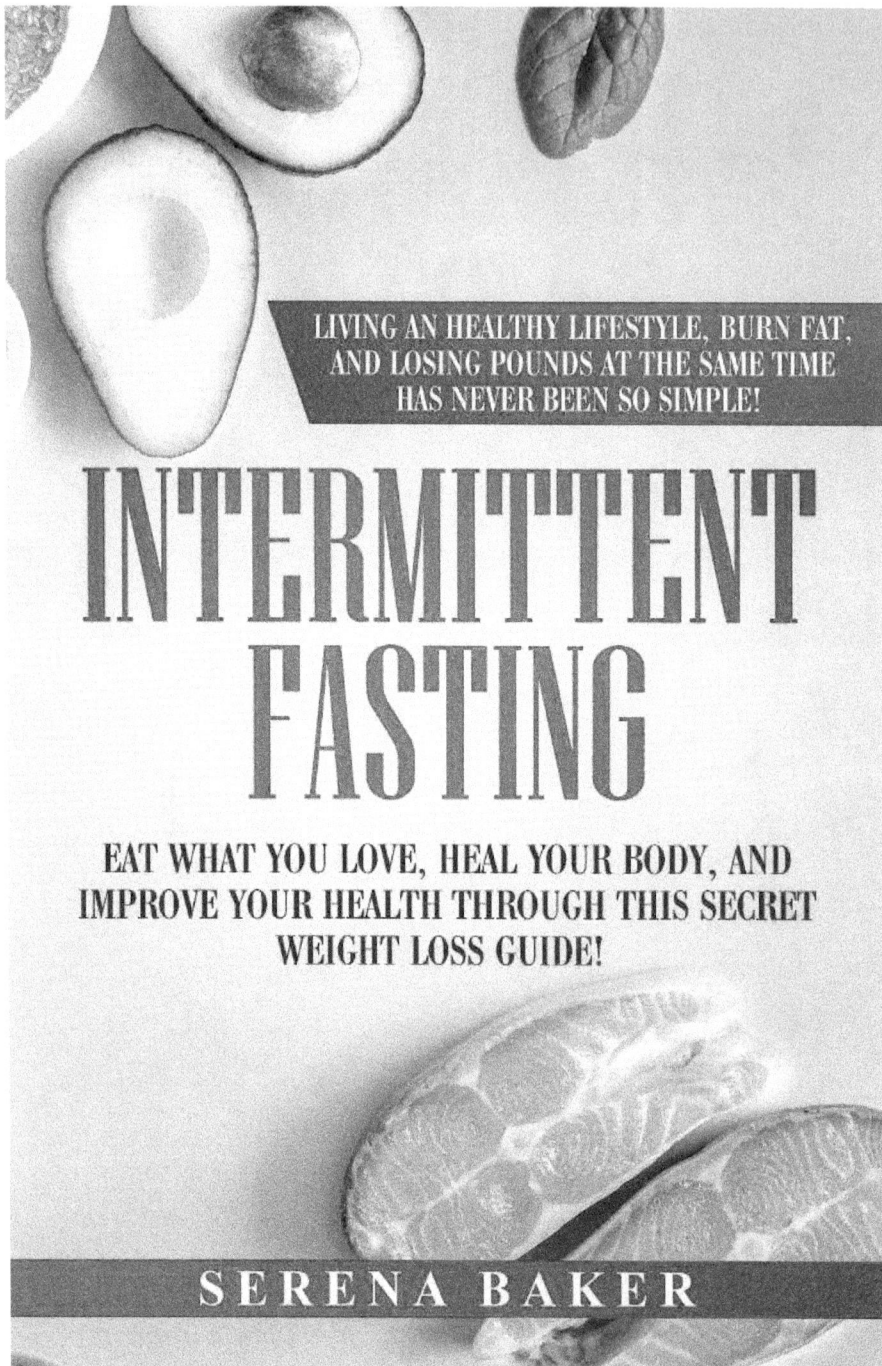

LIVING AN HEALTHY LIFESTYLE, BURN FAT, AND LOSING POUNDS AT THE SAME TIME HAS NEVER BEEN SO SIMPLE!

# INTERMITTENT FASTING

EAT WHAT YOU LOVE, HEAL YOUR BODY, AND IMPROVE YOUR HEALTH THROUGH THIS SECRET WEIGHT LOSS GUIDE!

## SERENA BAKER

# *Intermittent Fasting: The Guide*

*The best guide on Intermittent Fasting*

# Keto Fat
# BOMBS

COOKBOOK WITH 50 SWEET, SAVORY, AND FROZEN RECIPES TO SATISFY EVERY TASTE

BURN FAT AND ENJOY EVERY DESSERT, TREAT, OR OCCASION WITH THESE QUICK AND EASY LOW-CARB/HIGH-FAT SNACKS!

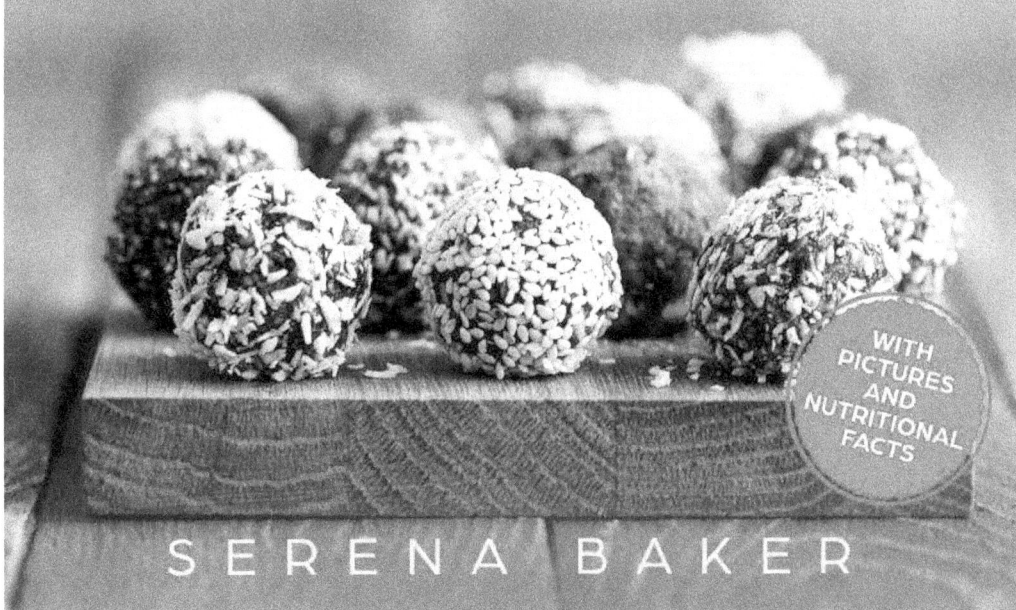

WITH PICTURES AND NUTRITIONAL FACTS

SERENA BAKER

## Keto Fat Bombs

*A collection of 50 mouthwatering keto recipes*

# Keto Diet for Beginners: The Guide

*The best guide on the Keto Diet*

# KETO
## Meal Prep

**QUICK, HEALTHY AND DELICIOUS
READY-TO-GO KETOGENIC DIET MEALS
TO PREP THAT ACTUALLY TASTE GOOD**

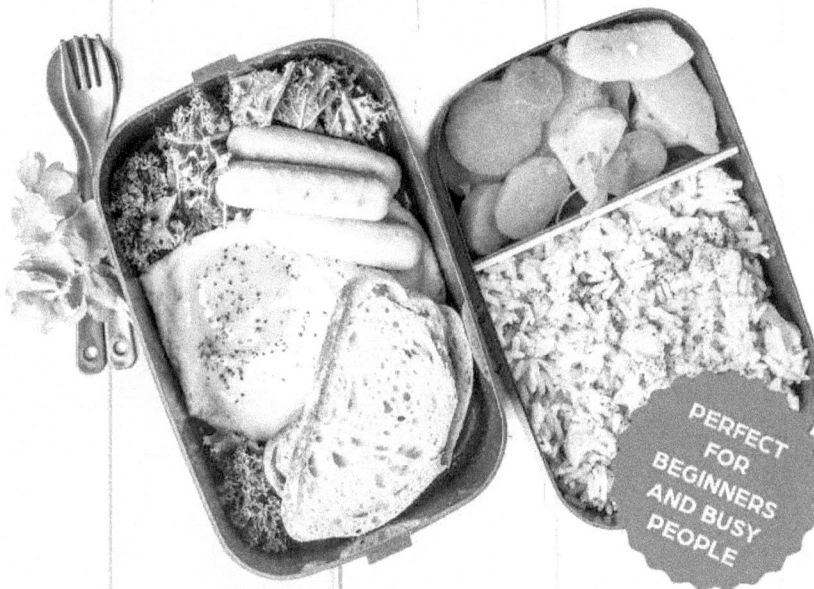

PERFECT
FOR
BEGINNERS
AND BUSY
PEOPLE

## SERENA BAKER

# *Keto Meal Prep*

*Healthy and delicious ketogenic diet meals to prep, grab, and go!*

# MEDITERRANEAN

# DIET

## *for beginners*

**FORM NEW MINI HABITS, INCREASE LONGEVITY, AND BURN FAT FOREVER WITH THE BEST SOLUTION TO A PALEO OR KETO DIET!**

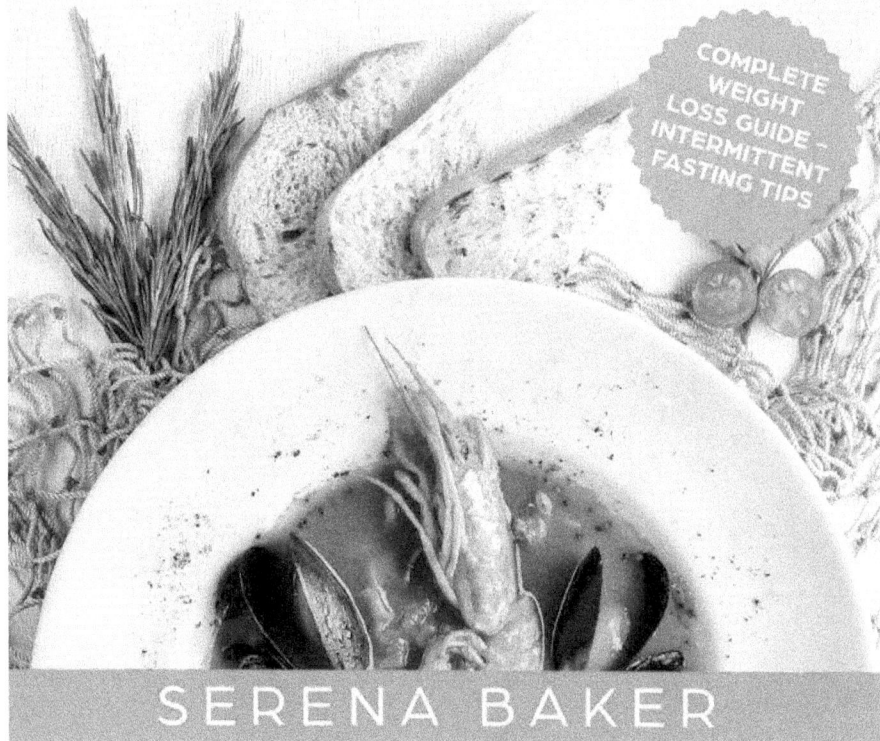

COMPLETE WEIGHT LOSS GUIDE – INTERMITTENT FASTING TIPS

## SERENA BAKER

# *Mediterranean Diet for Beginners: The Guide*

*The happiest diet on the planet*

CPSIA information can be obtained
at www.ICGtesting.com
Printed in the USA
LVHW060505261020
669798LV00009B/453